PROMOTING THE
HUMAN–ANIMAL BOND
IN
VETERINARY PRACTICE

SO .I. ES CENTRES

PROMOTING THE
HUMAN–ANIMAL BOND
IN
VETERINARY PRACTICE

Thomas E. Catanzaro, DVM, MHA, FACHE

Iowa State University Press / Ames

Thomas E. Catanzaro, DVM, MHA, FACHE, Diplomate, American College of Healthcare Executives, received his DVM from Colorado State University and his master's in healthcare administration from Baylor University. Dr. Catanzaro was the first veterinarian to receive board certification with the American College of Healthcare Executives. He is a charter member of the Delta Society, the original multi-disciplinary group studying human–animal–environment interactions; a charter member of the American Association of Human–Animal Bond Veterinarians; and a board member of VetOne, current advocates of the family–pet–veterinarian bond. In the last decade Catanzaro has visited, assisted, or consulted with over 1,400 veterinary practices. He is the author of a three-volume series, *Building the Successful Veterinary Practice,* published by Iowa State University Press, as well as six other books for the veterinary profession in the last three years.

© 2001 Iowa State University Press
All rights reserved

Iowa State University Press
2121 South State Avenue, Ames, Iowa 50014

Orders: 1-800-862-6657
Office: 1-515-292-0140
Fax: 515-292-3348
Web site: *www.isupress.com*

Authorization to photocopy items for internal or personal use, or the internal or personal use of specific clients, is granted by Iowa State University Press, provided that the base fee of $.10 per copy is paid directly to the Copyright Clearance Center, 222 Rosewood Drive, Danvers, MA 01923. For those organizations that have been granted a photocopy license by CCC, a separate system of payments has been arranged. The fee code for users of the Transactional Reporting Service is 0-8138-0382-9/2001$.10.

∞ Printed on acid-free paper in the United States of America

First edition, 2001

Library of Congress Cataloging-in-Publication Data

Catanzaro, Thomas E.
    Promoting the human-animal bond in veterinary practice / Thomas E. Catanzaro.—1st ed.
        p. cm.
    Includes bibliographical references.
    ISBN 0-8138-0382-9 (alk. paper)
    1. Veterinary medicine—Practice. 2. Human-animal relationships. 3. Veterinarian and client. I. Title.

SF756.4 .C37 2001
636.089'0696—dc21   2001016546

The last digit is the print number: 9 8 7 6 5 4 3 2 1

To Merlin

A head-butting buddy who was always glad to see me,
A silent meow, and a look was all that was needed;
I "scritched" his ears and he was happy, as was I.
He crossed the rainbow bridge last year, and I am still sad.

To Merlin, thanks for the memories.

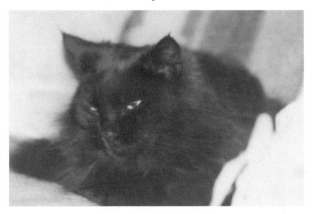

Contents

Related Works
by Dr. T.E. Catanzaro

AAHA Design Starter Kit for Veterinary Hospitals, 3rd edition. (with Gates Hafen Cochrane and John Knapp). 2000. Denver: AAHA.

Beyond the Successful Veterinary Practice: Succession Planning and Other Legal Issues. 2000. Ames: Iowa State University Press.

Building the Successful Veterinary Practice: Leadership Tools (volume 1). 1997. Ames: Iowa State University Press.

Building the Successful Veterinary Practice: Programs & Procedures (volume 2). 1998. Ames: Iowa State University Press. See chapter 2 for discussion of bonding clients and chapter 5 for a discussion of internal marketing.

Building the Successful Veterinary Practice: Innovation & Creativity (volume 3). 1998. Ames: Iowa State University Press. Discusses health alerts, new client newsletters, and other less common marketing concepts. Also includes the information on producing your own practice brochures mentioned in appendix T.

Death with Dignity—The Implications of Human/Animal Bond Interactions within the Hospice Programs. 1991. In *Universal Kinship—The Bond between All Living Things,* ed. Latham Foundation. Saratoga, CA: R & E Publishers.

Healthcare of the Well Pet. (with C. Jevring). 1998. Bailliere-Tindale. Review chapter 4, on the aging pet, to augment knowledge of thanatology.

A Study of the Human/Companion Animal Bond in Mobile Military Families in the United States. 1984. In *The Pet Connection: Its Influence on Our Health and Quality of Life,* ed. R.K. Anderson, B.L. Hart, and L.A. Hart. Minneapolis: Center to Study Human-Animal Relationships and Environments (CENSHARE), University of Minnesota.

Veterinary Healthcare Services: Options in Delivery (with T. Haig, P. Weinstein, J. Leake, and H. Howell). 2000. Ames: Iowa State University Press. See chapter 5 for discussion of "persuasion marketing." (See appendix W.) This text also supports the Preferred Client program presented in appendix C.

Veterinary Management in Transition: Preparing for the 21st Century. 2000. Ames: Iowa State University Press.

Veterinary Practice Management Secrets. (with P. Seibert, Jr.). 2000. Philadelphia: Lippicott/Hanley Belfus.

Preface

WHILE I am a Charter member of the Delta Society (circa 1980), a charter member of the American Association of Human-Animal Bond Veterinarians (circa 1990), and a board member of Vet-One (circa 1999), this book has been pending for over two decades. My initial human-animal bond family research was published in *The Pet Connection,* the CENSHARE (Center to Study Human-Animal Relationships and Environments, University of Minnesota) proceedings from early Delta Society meetings (circa 1983) in Minnesota and California. In 1982, following some preliminary Delta Society studies, I had developed a 32-question family survey; this survey was distributed at 63 military veterinary facilities across the United States, and 961 of 1500 surveys were completed and returned (64 percent response rate). Concurrently I had surveyed the veterinarians in those facilities and asked them to predict their clients' responses; there were 86 veterinarians who responded (50.2 percent response rate). The responses of those veterinarians were published in JAVMA in 1988 (Vol. 192, No. 12, June 15, 1988), and while they understood the professional and scientific values of their clients, they often underestimated the social interdependence between client and pet. This bias has remained unchanged in many practices during the last decade.

Dr. Leo Bustad committed his life and his golden years to promoting the importance of the human-animal bond, supported since the beginning by Linda Hines, the current president/CEO of the Delta Society. Many caring individuals have spent over two decades promoting the bond; healthcare professionals like Tom Lane, Bill and Michael McCulloch, John Neu, Earl Strimple, Lynn Anderson, Hiram Kitchin, Kathy Mitchner, Bill Kay, Lynnette and Ben Hart, James Harris, Erwin Small, R. K. Anderson, Marv Samuelson, and many more that space prohibits listing. In more recent years, younger, compassionate professionals like Marty Becker, Greg Ogilvie, Chuck Wayner, and others in "Vet One" have taken up the challenge to establish the human-animal bond as part of every veterinary healthcare delivery program.

This work is designed to express the compassionate aspects of the human-animal bond in practical implementation terms for the veterinary practice team to embrace and for healthcare professionals to pursue with commitment. The human-animal bond is so obvious to most veterinary practice team members that it is often overlooked as being an integral program to routinely assess and improve. It is hoped that this volume will assist practices in committing the attention and resources needed to ensure the client bond, thereby establishing a greater patient return rate, which translates into "good business" in this new millennium of veterinary healthcare delivery.

Thomas E. Catanzaro, DVM, MHA, FACHE
Diplomate, American College of Healthcare Executives

Introduction

THE HUMAN-ANIMAL bond can be traced back to the earliest days of civilization, but only in the past couple decades have pets become accepted as "companion" animals. The people who raised you taught you pet care . . . and you probably said, "I'll never raise kids the way I was raised!" Most people have not had comprehensive courses on being stewards of other living entities, whether it be animals or children. It is our job as veterinary professionals to understand the differences and help clients become better stewards of animals. The client/animal owner categories are shown in Table I.1 on the next page.

To begin this text, we need to look at the beginnings of the human-animal bond (HAB) study process. I started studying the human-animal bond immediately after the 1980 Delta Society organizational Meeting at Pennsylvania; Leo Bustad's vision has had a lasting impact on me. As a strong scouter, I started the process by studying family values, and I used the transient military communities as a sample base. In August 1982, the military human–companion animal bond survey was developed. It focused on a cross section of American pet owners, the mobile military family group; the pet's role in the quality of life of service members; and the pet's role in community health. The baseline concepts

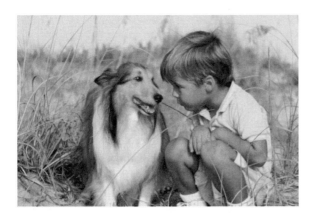

were developed from Dr. Ann Cain's 1977 62-family survey, "A Study of Pets in the Family System" (Cain 1981). The survey questions were developed from the subjective responses to the Cain study, then expanded based on the professional healthcare experience of the military veterinarians, social workers, and psychiatric officers at the U.S. Army Health Services Command.

Table I.1. Client–animal owner categories

Traits	D Clients: Do Only the "Required"	C/B Clients: Preventive Care Is Consideration for Owner	A/B Clients: Does Most Anything Needed as Steward of Another
Owner treats pet like:	An animal	Family	A child
Human-animal bond	No awareness	Aware	Significant importance
Pet's health and well-being	Low	Moderate	Optimal
Pet's happiness	Not a concept	Concern in general	Important every day
Pet's life expectancy	Variable	Medium	High
Rewards owner receives from pet	Low awareness	Moderate awareness	Optimal
Clinic's economic return and client-base growth	Volume required	Mid-range productivity	High return rate productivity
Emotional rewards for hospital staff	Strained	Mid-road	Peace of mind
Overall impact on future success of the veterinary profession	Damaging	Status quo	Leaders in the community

To properly analyze the mobile population's opinions of human–companion animal bond factors, 1500 copies of a 10-page, 32-question survey were distributed to 63 military installations; 961 surveys were returned (64%). The effects of human-animal interaction on community, family, and animal health have an extensive impact upon the military member, the military installation, and the military healthcare delivery system. Results showed significant sociological and psychological factors that influence the quality of life of the mobile military member and his/her family. To date, there have been many subsequent studies, but this one has had the most significant N and has been validated at most every opportunity. Family values about companion animals have not changed; they have just been allowed to surface.

Concurrent with the client survey, a lateral survey was conducted on the question of how well veterinarians can predict their clients' human-animal bond, and the results were very revealing.

In the survey of 63 military veterinary facilities, responses from 961 clients were compared with the predictions of the clients' responses by the 86 servicing U.S. Army Veterinary Corps practitioners. Results revealed both sociological and psychological factors that influenced the quality of life of mobile military members and their families. The survey also revealed that, whereas newly graduated veterinarians understood the professional and scientific values of their clients, they often underestimated the social interdependence between client and pet. The military veterinarians contacted in this survey were considered representative of the new graduate, and the results were relevant to any civilian practitioner concerned with client relations or hiring new graduates.

The primary goal of the original study compared here was to identify the benefits of companion animals to those that have accepted stewardship for them. This comparison was laterally completed by the attending veterinarians in hopes of providing information that might increase the sensitivity of educators and veterinarians to the importance of the human–companion animal bond in client relations.

Methods and Materials

Baseline concepts were developed from a 62-family survey. Survey questions were developed from the subjective responses to that family survey; then the questions were expanded on the basis of the professional healthcare experience of the military veterinarians, social workers, and psychiatry officers at the U.S. Army Health Services Command. The questionnaire was refined into a 32-question, computer-ready format. To initiate the survey, 1500 copies of the military human–companion animal bond survey were distributed to 63 military installations; 961 client surveys were returned (64%). Also, it was requested that the supporting military veterinarian complete a survey and attempt to predict the average client's response; estimates were received from 86 veterinarians (50.2% response by veterinarians). The distribution of the client survey was conducted so that every person that walked through the door on a given morning was handed a survey and asked to complete it to the best of their ability.

The typical military veterinary facility (referred to as an Animal Disease Prevention and Control Facility) operates by appointment only, for approximately 12 to 16 composite hours during a week. The veterinarian was usually a new graduate, with the values, attitudes, and skills that had accumulated after four years of veterinary medical education. During the remainder of duty time (30 or more hours per week), the military veterinarian is scheduled to do community public health activities, such as sanitary inspections, zoonotic disease surveillance, hospital committee attendance, or supervision of enlisted personnel who do food inspection. Clients of the Department of Defense and the scope of services are unique in that failure to register an animal can cause an owner to be severely punished.

Most veterinary facilities on military installations are only permitted to conduct diagnostic procedures until the causative agent is identified. If a zoonotic or economically significant disease is identified or if an organism that causes the spread of a potentially zoonotic organism is suspected and the acute condition can be readily cured, the veterinarian may treat the animal. However, if a non-zoonotic condition is diagnosed or treatment would require long-term care, it is requested that the facility refer the case. For these diagnostic and vaccination services, the average client paid fees approximate to the large format retailers (LFRs) in the area (approximately 24% of military clients are eligible for food stamps).

The art of veterinary medicine has been defined in many ways, but for the sake of this discussion, it will be defined as the veterinarian's ability to detect the client's bond with his/her pet and to predict how that bond may influence the decision process on patient care. Respondents were asked to place an X on a line below the words (Always, Usually, Sometimes, Never) most usually representing their feelings.

Always   Usually   Sometimes   Never
   | | | |
   _____

This format was used throughout the survey to better identify the trends. Accuracy was increased by dividing the line into at least 10 segments when quantifying the responses for computer tabulation. Exceptional ratings were required to be on the left or right 20% of the line; responses marked on the center 60% were considered neutral.

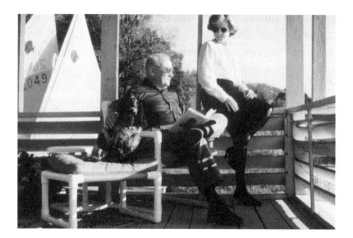

Results

The respondents in the owner survey population consisted of 34.2% husbands, 52.9% wives, and 12.9% other, ranging in age from 19 to 71. The veterinarians responding were predominantly male (83%) and were within the first three years after their graduation from veterinary school. The sample sizes were considered adequate to compensate for particular practice irregularities or great variances in responses. The client survey showed that 77.4% visited their veterinarians two or more times per year per pet (compared with 70.9%, as estimated by the veterinarians); 59.8% were exceptionally satisfied with the veterinary services (veterinarians thought only 3.2% would be exceptionally satisfied); 34.4% usually celebrated the pet's birthday (veterinarians predicted 17.4%); 53.1% displayed pictures of their pet at home (compared with 44.2% as estimated by the veterinarians); and 50.4% stated their pet was extremely important to their family (the veterinarians predicted only 26.7% would rate pets this high on the importance scale).

Questions were included in an attempt to quantify the reasons why an animal was less important to some persons. Housing limitations were ranked by clients and veterinarians as the most frequent reason for nonownership; inconvenience was ranked second by both; client reason number 3 was too much time required for care (veterinarians rated this 8 on a scale of 10); and client reason number 10 was undesirable behavior (veterinarians estimated this would be number 6).

The veterinarians predicted that 23.8% would spend $100 or more per year per pet for other than food, but 37.8% of the clients reported that they spent $100 or more. The veterinarian and client responses agreed on what children gained from being associated with a pet; in order of most important to least, these were learning responsibility, companionship, pleasure, respect for life, gentleness, and education in life processes.

In evaluating the changes associated with bringing a pet into a household, the survey addressed family interaction changes. The factors and changes are shown in Table I.2. A better comparison was expected when discussing potential animal problem areas; however, Table I.3 shows this was not the case.

To evaluate why certain people used certain veterinarians, 14 reasons for using their current civilian veterinarian were provided and respondents were asked to rate them in order of importance (Table I.4), with 1 being most important and 14 being least important . Veterinarians predicted well the reasons for selection of a practice, but their estimates of the importance of a pet diverged largely from the responses of the clients. When clients were asked to evaluate how important their pet was to their family, 50.3% reported extremely important, 33.8% very important, and 12.4% important; veterinarians predicted approximately half this response rate. To better evaluate the importance of the companion animal, the line scale was used for 12 specific situations (see Table I.5).

In addition to questions concerning the importance of the pet to the family, other questions were posed to evaluate the anthropomorphic tendencies of the respondents. When asked how the companion animal fit into the family, 68.3% of the clients stated that the pet had full family member status, whereas only 38.4% of the veterinarians predicted this degree of bonding. Later in the survey, the questions were rephrased and the client was asked whether the pet was afforded people status in the family. The line scale was used and the respondent was asked to rate the status from always through usually and sometimes to never. The results showed 38.8% of the clients believed their pet was always afforded people status (veterinarians predicted 16.3%), 71.7% believed their pets were usually to always afforded people status (veterinarians predicted 52.3%), and 3% reported that their pet was never afforded people status (veterinarians predicted 8.1%).

Table I.2. Changes in family interaction with the introduction of a pet

Increase (%)			Decrease (%)	
Clients' Response	Veterinarians' Prediction	Family Factor	Clients' Response	Veterinarians' Prediction
8.0	12.8	Arguing	9.2	9.3
59.3	54.7	Affection expressed around pet	0.7	0.0
6.8	1.2	Travel and freedom	39.3	55.8
70.1	65.1	Happiness and fun	1.4	0.0
63.5	68.6	Responsibility	0.7	0.0
51.7	44.8	Time together as family (with pet)	1.3	2.3

Table I.3. Expected problems associated with pet ownership

More Than Expected (%)			Less Than Expected (%)	
Clients' Response	Veterinarians' Prediction	Problem Area	Clients' Response	Veterinarians' Prediction
15.1	36.0	Housebreaking	31.5	15.1
17.8	32.6	Disciplining	27.0	12.8
6.4	9.3	Feeding	23.7	15.1
10.6	17.4	Behavior with family	22.2	18.6
11.9	29.1	Location or territory	19.7	10.5
18.1	30.2	Grooming	17.1	12.8
14.5	27.9	Cleaning	16.7	10.5

Many traits or attributes are credited to the companion animal during daily conversations, so the survey asked specifically what special characteristics the pet displayed within the family. The responses were placed on the line scale, as shown in Table I.6. In evaluating the responsiveness of the pet within the family, clients reported usually quick positive responses 86% of the time for parents and 48% of the time for children, whereas the veterinarians estimated 89% for parents and 62% for children. To consider negative interactions, the question

Table I.4. Reasons for clients selecting a civilian veterinarian

Reason	Clients' Response	Veterinarians' Prediction
Range or scope of services	1	1
Professional skills of veterinarian	2	6
Availability of after-hours service	3	2
Convenience to residence	4	3
Appointment hours	5	4
Personality of veterinarian	6	5
Telephone assistance	7	9
Cost of services	8	11
Personality of staff	9	7
Veterinary specialists on staff	10	10
Facility appearance	11	8
House call services availability	12	14
Knowledge of unique problems	13	13
Parking	14	12

Table I.5. Evaluation of the importance of the pet in specific situations

Great Importance (%)			No Importance (%)	
Clients' Response	Veterinarians' Prediction	Situation	Clients' Response	Veterinarians' Prediction
75.4	46.5	At all times	1.7	1.2
73.2	58.1	Temporary absence of spouse	6.7	2.3
71.4	46.5	Free time or relaxation	2.8	1.2
69.6	66.3	Childhood period	9.7	2.3
68.4	67.4	Sad, lonely, depressed	5.1	3.5
58.6	47.7	Marriage without children	25.5	15.1
53.3	32.6	Temporary absence of children	17.5	14.0
52.1	44.2	During illness or after other's death	14.0	7.0
50.4	45.3	During crisis or separation or divorce	16.4	8.1
48.2	23.3	During moves or relocations	17.6	15.1
44.5	27.9	Teenage period	16.1	9.3
35.7	23.3	Unemployment	31.4	24.4

Note: The percentages on each line are of the total population and show those that recorded their X on the right or left 20% of the answer line; the percentage unaccounted for was in the center 60%, considered neutral for this study.

was rephrased, and 23% of the respondents reported usually quick negative responses to the parents and 25% toward the children. The veterinarians estimated 30% usually quick negative responses toward the parents and 29% toward

Table I.6. Reported special characteristics shown by companion animals

Great Display of Trait (%)			No Display of Trait (%)	
Clients' Response	Veterinarians' Prediction	Characteristic	Clients' Response	Veterinarians' Prediction
89.4	82.6	Greets you upon coming home	1.5	1.2
77.0	58.1	Pet understands when you talk to him/her	0.9	1.2
73.0	60.5	Communicates to you	1.4	3.5
59.6	51.2	Demand for attention	2.3	3.5
59.3	48.8	Understands or is sensitive to your moods	4.2	5.8
49.7	27.9	Stays close when you're anxious or upset	10.7	18.6
44.9	31.4	Sleeps with family member	34.8	37.2
22.6	20.9	Mimics your emotions	23.4	30.2
11.8	16.3	Hides or withdraws when you are anxious or upset	56.3	38.4
10.6	10.5	Expresses feelings that you cannot or do not	58.6	41.9
3.9	7.0	Develops illness when family tension is high	84.3	70.0

Note: The percentages on each line are of the total population, and show those that recorded their X on the right or left 20% of the answer line; the percentage unaccounted for was in the center 60%, considered neutral for this study.

the children. Respondents reported about half the pets never showed a quick negative response to adults, whereas the veterinarians estimated that only one-third would never show a quick negative response. Clients reported that less than 1% of the pets never showed a quick positive response, and veterinarians basically agreed by estimating that all pets would show a quick positive response at some time.

A question was posed concerning the pet's response when family members showed affection toward each other. The clients reported that 78.7% of the pets wanted active involvement (veterinarians estimated 68.6%), whereas 6.8% of the pets never responded (veterinarians estimated 9.3% would never respond). When asked about the pet's response during times of high anxiety or crisis within the family, 59.2% of the owners reported their pet usually wanted interaction with the family, whereas the veterinarians estimated only 37.2% would want interaction. The companion animal's response to a new addition in the family group was surveyed; 38.3% of the family animals showed positive behavior changes, whereas only 16.3% showed negative behavior changes, with 45.4% showing no change. The veterinarians predicted only 15.1% would show positive change, 12.8% would show a negative change, and 72.1% would show no

Table I.7. Expected disposition of animal when family relocates

| Move Within Country (%) | | | Move Overseas (%) | |
Clients' Response	Veterinarians' Prediction	Action	Clients' Response	Veterinarians' Prediction
65.4	82.9	Take with you to new home	35.6	20.0
13.3	11.8	Ship to new home	46.8	49.2
5.2	3.9	Give away	8.9	20.0
1.5	1.3	Turn in for adoption	2.8	9.2
1.6	—	Give to Humane Society	1.4	1.5
1.1	—	Sell	1.4	—
1.1	—	Turn in for veterinary disposal	1.0	—
1.0	—	Release to farm or woodland		0.7
0.9	—	Abandon	0.8	

Table I.8. Expected client action when pet becomes seriously ill

Situational Response	Clients' Response	Veterinarians' Prediction
Do whatever the military veterinarian recommended	41.2	29.9
Do whatever was needed if pet could be returned to normal health	19.8	13.4
Do whatever was needed for disabled pet as long as no pain or suffering	18.1	11.8
Do whatever the civilian veterinarian recommended	10.6	15.3
Have pet euthanized if treatment costs more than $200 to $250	6.0	18.1
Have pet euthanized before treatment costs any more	1.8	6.7
Let nature take its course	1.3	1.9
Replace ailing pet with healthy pet	0.3	3.5

change in behavior. The pet's role as a third party in arguments or in stress relief was surveyed by the question, "When tension between two persons exceeds a certain level, it has been noted that a third party is brought into the discussion to dissipate the intensity of the tension; does this occur with your pet becoming that third party?" The survey revealed that 8.2% of the respondents said the pet was always the third party involved, 43.8% reported that it occurred sometimes to always, and 38.4% reported that it never occurred. The veterinarians estimated it would occur always in 2.5% of the cases, sometimes to always in 46.9%, and never in 28.4%.

With the highly mobile, fast food lifestyle seen in today's work place, it was thought to be important to ask what would happen to the pet at times of family relocations or household moves. The scope of choices and responses are shown in Table I.7. To further evaluate the strength of the family-pet bond, respondents were asked what they would do if their pet became seriously ill; the results are shown in Table I.8.

Respondents were asked to describe the degree of loss felt by the family if they had ever had a pet that was lost, had died, or was killed. Almost all clients reported important to extreme loss (94.4%), and 58.8% of those said it was an extreme loss; only 0.1% of the clients reported no loss was felt. Whereas the veterinarians' estimate for important to extreme loss approximated the clients' (93.8%), they said only 27.2% would feel an extreme loss; also, the veterinarians estimated no client would report no loss felt. Another questions was asked dealing with the disposition of the deceased companion animal, and the results are shown in Table I.9. Almost 70% of the clients wished to bury their animal in some way.

Table I.9. Preferred companion animal remains disposition methods

Disposition Action	Clients' Response	Veterinarians' Prediction
Bury in marked grave, but not in pet cemetery	42.6	34.6
Take to veterinarian or humane society for disposal	28.3	27.2
Bury, but not anywhere special	14.8	27.1
Bury with full ceremony in pet cemetery	2.8	6.2
Let someone else dispose of pet	1.6	1.2
Dispose of by standard waste removal services	0.7	3.7

Discussion

The proximity of the Animal Disease Prevention and Control Facility enhances the choice of military clients to use the military veterinarian. Although the client pays for all goods received, there is a perception of true value because high profit should not be a motive of the military facility operations. The facility operates to protect the health of the soldier and the public health of the federal community surrounding the military working/training environment; the clients accept the restricted (by appointment only, refer if chronic) veterinary medical service support program as necessary for typical military readiness and mobilization necessities.

Conversely, a newly graduated military veterinarian and a newly graduated civilian-salaried veterinarian are expected to have similar value profiles. A new graduate brings only knowledge learned in school and a small amount of personal experience learned from another veterinarian. A new veterinarian enters an established practice with established rules, procedures, and client handling techniques; the new practitioner must comply to the practice standards already established. A recent graduate generally requires close supervision and development in areas of client relations.

The differences in veterinarian prediction and client response shown in Table I.2 were attributed to the youth of the military veterinarians, especially in reference to their family experiences. It was expected that Table I.3 would show better predictions, but the great "less than expected" response by owners surprised the surveyors also.

The veterinarian was pessimistic about responses of pets to family interactions, generally predicting significant negative responses that were not reported by clients. The clients reported that less than 1% of the pets never showed a quick positive response, and the veterinarians supported this inherent belief that all animals have some good in them.

The responses in Table I.8 attack the disposable pet concepts so common in low income clientele. The figures reflected a responsible pet ownership being supported by disbelieving veterinarians.

There are emotional stresses that occur when a pet becomes lost, dies, or is killed, and Table I.9 was designed to compare client values to common practice methods. In theory, clients and veterinarians were equally sensitive to the need for burial, but we need to question then why cremation is so often recommended.

Results of the survey implied military pet owners have more intense human-animal bond feelings than other groups in similar surveys. It appeared that the economic, educational, and social structure of the military respondent were the key factors affecting results of the survey. In this survey population, 54% were mothers, less than 34% had a college education, and most earned less than $20,000 per year. In all comparable studies, the respondents were better educated, included more females, or had a higher economic status in the surveyed population. Also, identifying the center 60% of the response line as neutral allowed the intensity of the clients' emotions to be better identified; this also caused the responding veterinarians to appear less perceptive. The veterinarian estimated the client effectively in matters of professional or scientific judgment but appeared to underestimate the intensity of the social interdependence between animal and man. If the negative responses were evaluated for the same answer line, it would be noted that the veterinarians generally overestimated the response; that is, they could not imagine clients who couldn't see the value of a companion animal. Veterinarians' responses often were on the center 60% of the answer line, thereby masking their mediated response. When the educational trends toward teaching ethics and values are observed, (Talbot 1983, McCulloch et al. 1983) it can be seen that universities are well aware of the needs, as is the American Veterinary Medical Association. But when these ethics are applied, the new graduate appears to mediate his response from his intense personal beliefs. From management experience, this response could be credited to a new employee syndrome, common to the military and civilian practice; that is, what will the boss tolerate?

Whereas the family importance of the companion animal appeared substantially greater in this survey population, than in populations considered in other surveys, the responses concerning companion animals in family situations were similar in most populations. The low estimate by the veterinarians might be indicative of a lack of experience or of memories of a few bad experiences in the first few years of practice. Regardless of cause, the importance of the human–companion animal bond in client relations must be realized, and sensitivities should be increased in both academic and practice environments.

The perceptions reflected in the above study have been indicative of most veterinary practices visited during the delivery of our veterinary consulting services (over 1400 in the past 14 years). The 26 practice program appendices offered here CANNOT all be implemented at once; the practice leadership needs to select and implement one at a time. The Delta Society (800-869-6898) has provided many of the pictures for this text and, as the international clearing house for human-animal bond studies and information, has more program resources than any practice could ever hope to implement; this is an important group to join and utilize in the fast changing world of community-based veterinary practice.

It is my sincere hope that the veterinary reader will embrace the simple fact that the human-animal bond is why we are here, that our veterinary healthcare delivery programs must be founded in solid patient advocacy, and that the values that bring clients and staff into our sphere of influence provide a charter of delivery excellence that must be caring, compassionate, and nurturing. This profession is more of a "calling" than any other healthcare profession, and our patients must trust us more than any other patient in any other healthcare field. The trust of a patient and his/her steward cannot be violated with discounts, bait-and-switch programs, or a "buyer beware" mentality. We each must hold ourselves to a higher authority and to a higher standard; we must speak for the animal's well being and protect the covenant that goes back to the beginning of civilization. Our profession must stand tall and be counted when issues of animal welfare are being discussed. We must be leaders in the human-animal bond awareness efforts of our society.

References

Catanzaro, T.E. 1984. A Study of the Human/Companion Animal Bond in Mobile Military Families in the United States. In *The Pet Connection: Its Influence on Our Health and Quality of Life,* ed. R.K. Anderson, B.L. Hart, and L.A. Hart. Minneapolis: Center to Study Human-Animal Relationships and Environments (CENSHARE), University of Minnesota.

Cain, A.O. 1981. A Study of Pets in the Family System. Paper presented at the first International Conference on the Human–Companion Animal Bond, Philadelphia, PA, October.

Charles, Charles and Associates. 1983. The Veterinary Services Market: Study Summary and Report on Promoting Veterinary Services. Overland Park, KS.

Horn, J.C., and J. Meer. 1984. The Pleasure of Their Company, *Psychology Today,* August, 52–58.

Anderson, R.K., B.L. Hart, and L.A. Hart (eds.). 1984. *The Pet Connection: Its Influence on Our Health and Quality of Life.* Minneapolis: Center to Study Human-Animal Relationships and Environments (CENSHARE), University of Minnesota.

Hopkins, A.F. 1978. Ethical Implications in Issues and Decisions in Companion Animal Medicine. In *Implications of History and Ethics to Medicine-Veterinary and Human,* L.B. McCulloch and J.P. Morris, eds. College Station: Texas A&M University Press.

Talbot, R.B. 1983. Exploring Ethical and Value Issues in Veterinary Medicine. *Journal of Veterinary Medicine Education* (8th Symposium) 9(3).

McCulloch, W.F., N.D. Heidelbaugh, L.M. Hines, and L.K. Bustad. 1983. The Human-Animal Bond in the Public Health Curriculum. *Journal of the American Veterinary Medical Association* 183(12).

McCulloch, W.F. 1985. The Veterinarian's Education about the Human-Animal bond and Animal-Facilitated Therapy. *The Veterinary Clinics of North America, Small Animal Practice.* 15(2).

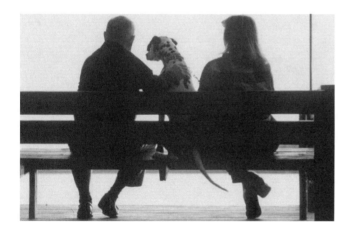

PROMOTING THE

HUMAN–ANIMAL BOND

IN

VETERINARY PRACTICE

1

Bonding the Client to Your Practice

TODAY WE are told we must work smarter, not harder. Some consultants have their favorite solution: "Give me your current office call and I can set your prices to the appropriate level that will increase your net" . . . or . . . "Profit centers must be developed" . . . or . . . "This new equipment/system will save you money in the long run" . . . or . . . "Send your people to this school/seminar to increase your profits" . . . or . . . "Subscribe to this newsletter for all the management answers." Regardless of the consultant pitch, the unspoken bottom line is, "good medicine is good business."

Good Medicine in the Practice

Good medicine is what we were trained to provide. Yet, somehow the day-to-day crush of practice squeezes the professional juices from our treatment plan. Couldn't happen to you? Try this quick test: Pull the first five records from any position in the first half of your hospital patient files (the "S" file is in the last half and has been overused already). Now systematically review each record for your patient advocacy. Here are some questions to ask:

- Were vaccinations, fecal, heartworm testing/FELV offered and/or recorded at the first contact?
- Does every client leave with a Recheck/Recall/Reminder entry (every client meets at least one of the three Rs).
- Did the following visit note some form of resolution of the previous problem(s)?
- Can you determine how many animals are in the household, and is there a separate record for every patient in the household?
- How often are dental grades recorded and/or dentals recommended?
- Are there sequential weights recorded for *every* animal, has each been quantified with a "body score," and what have been the actions when there have been weight changes?
- What is the *consistent* pain management program that emerges on review; are there recurring pain scores for all inpatient cases?
- How is risk assessment of anesthesia candidates recorded and what is the practice consistency on preanesthetic laboratory screening?

- Can the practice's imaging philosophy be established by the presenting complaint review; is there a diagnostic consistency for grade 3+ dentals, limping, chronic gut problems, moist rales, cardiac murmurs, and similar positive indications for imaging?
- Are client refusals or deferrals recorded?
- Are handouts noted on the record so we remember which ones we have explained? No handout should ever be given without some form of personalized professional overview of the subject.
- Were all the previous medications given for the full duration and did they work?
- Can you determine if a client who hasn't been back "on time" has been contacted?
- Do other animals in the same household get prophylactic treatments?
- Do we catch up records on all pets belonging to a client at every visit?

How many times have you found yourself making excuses because the above answers were less than professionally satisfying?

Patient Advocacy

> *Advocate: one who pleads the cause of another.*
> —Webster's Dictionary

I have found it much more difficult to teach a practice staff internal marketing than to help them become patient advocates. We no longer talk in "shoulds" or "recommendations"; rather, we speak in terms of "need," as in, "Fluffy needs to be tested for heartworms after your winter vacation down south." At the same time, we need to infuse our staff with respect for the client to waive any needed treatment. Waivers are recorded, occasionally with their initials just to reinforce the severity of the need, right after the plan in the medical record.

Good medicine starts when the client makes the first phone call (answered within three rings). Good medicine means never putting someone on hold without their verbal consent. Good medicine means for each veterinarian every fifth appointment space is left blank for same-day emergency services ("E" annotation or shaded space). Good medicine means an emergency as perceived by the client, not by the receptionist. If unused, the "E" space becomes catch-up time, a coffee-break rest period, a recall, or just a time to observe the rest of the team delivering quality healthcare.

Good medicine means introducing yourself upon entering the room, and touching the animal early. Only nerds lean against the wall, cross their arms, and question the client at length while the animal is suffering (in the client's opinion). You only have three to four minutes before your body language makes the client decide on your concern. Is your reception area a "waiting room," or has it been a good client experience where smiles and concerns have "hosted" the client into the exam room? If you teach yourself to listen to a client (not just hear what they are saying), you will be able to detect the concern, frustration, anxiety, or maybe even confidence in what they are saying. As you examine the pet, do you convey the good news (the specific normals, the good care) or do you silently skim the animal and give just an overall "okay" at the end? Clients enjoy hearing that the eyes are clear, the bladder feels normal, the intestines palpate healthy, the coat is glossy, the lungs are clear, both ears are clean, or whatever.

Does your receptionist offer to reschedule late arriving clients or on-time clients when your "schedule has been interrupted" (don't ever just "run late")? Many clients would rather come back for a different appointment after they do a few more errands than wait for 45 minutes while you catch up.

Look at the first impression the client sees. The curb appeal, the dog access/relief areas, and the first impression of the receiving desk all set the tone for the visit. Look at the reception room. Can a nervous cat and owner find a corner for protection? Can a lady safely tie her dog while she goes to the rest room? Are your displays framed (or do you just tape things to the wall like a teenager)? Neatness counts. Brightness and cheer have led to open receiving desks, bright wallpaper, and smiles. The days of dark paneling and small windows for "plush luxury" have yielded to "bright and cheerful." Old magazines are not needed in the reception area. There are many quality handouts and booklets available for free that can be read. Behind the scenes scrapbooks, practice client/pet scrapbooks, or even the *Delta Society Journal* can also be made available.

Good medicine means you are really concerned with the three Rs (recheck, reminder, recall). If a client does not return for the recheck at the prescribed time, you initiate a recall. The "Doctor and I" format has worked very successfully. The technician or receptionist automatically initiates the recall as needed. Introducing themselves, the veterinary facility, and then the question, "The Doctor and I were wondering (1) since we didn't see you this week if everything is okay" . . . or . . . (2) "whether you had any questions now that you have been home a few days" . . . or . . . (3) "if you think Fluffy needs more medication." When the response is other than what a paraprofessional can handle, the technician or receptionist can always say, "That's something the doctor would be concerned about. She/he reserves time for client phone calls between 6 and 8 *(or 1 and 3 if your hospital has a slow midday)*. Will you be home at that time?"

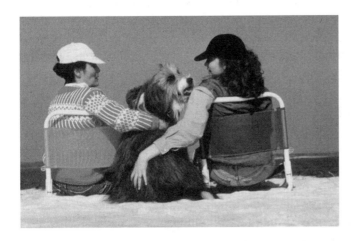

If you don't have time set aside daily for veterinarian callbacks, establish the time now. You can't afford to be on-call to the telephone, or out-of-touch all day.

Putting It to the Test

It all translates to patient advocacy, doing what is needed for the health and welfare of the animal. Good medicine is simply doing what is needed. Allowing the client the right to decide to waive the needed care will yield far more net than deciding for clients that they can't afford something. While our net is not a reason to be a patient advocate, it can be seen as an acceptable reward for good medicine and high professional standards for healthcare delivery.

The human–companion animal bond is hard to measure, but we can recognize it when we see it. Patient advocacy is a nice philosophy, but it also seems hard to measure. If we can't measure it, we can't manage it. We need to look at an indicator that will work for most practices.

Build a patient advocacy factor chart. It needs to be on the same monthly horizontal axis as any other monthly fiscal chart so it can be compared for relationships. The vertical axis is practice specific and is derived by taking the total monthly income and dividing it by an annual visit factor (e.g., the number of rabies vaccinations given in that same month). If your practice is in a three-year vaccination area, you may consider using the annual "distemper" vaccination or the "annual physical" rate in lieu of the rabies vaccinations. This method of charting gives you a feeling for the annual value of the animal to the practice.

This patient advocacy factor concept can be better understood through a practical application. We all know what happens to the average monthly client transaction fee when over-the-counter sales increase. It goes down. Now try this return trade concept using the patient advocacy factor chart. Increases in over-the-counter sales for the good of the pet will cause the graph to go up. If this graph line is tracking on an upward trend, even if your average transaction charge is staying level or dropping, it means clients are coming in more often, possibly for smaller purchases per time. Usually, the return clients are spending far more at the practice per year, so be happy!

Which tracking system would motivate your staff to try harder to be a patient advocate? Which system better monitors the more frequently returning client? Which is a better indicator of full service? Which is a better reflection of good medicine? Which veterinary healthcare delivery approach recognizes the value of the human-animal bond at the level of the client's perceptions?

Bonding the Client to Your Practice

In this day of a veterinarian on virtually every corner, the average client has two or more veterinary practices within 15 minutes of their home. It is likely that our better clients even drive past one or two practices just to get to "their veterinarian." It is this type of bond that must be developed as we build a practice, and it starts by the entire staff becoming aware that the human–companion animal bond is the basis of a caring practice philosophy. The chart below provides some new nomenclature for this new practice culture:

Acquiring a dog may be the only opportunity
a human ever has to choose a relative.

As our veterinary practices develop new ways of talking to our clients, remember to stress the verbal culture change within your staff that is needed to change their traditional mind set:

• Resort managers, not kennel masters
• Animal caretakers/pet partners, not kennel kids
• Comfort rooms, not empty exam rooms
• Whelping center suites/not large runs
• Hospice care suites, not large runs; a nursing/hospitalization alternative to boarding
• VIP (very important pet) suites, not large runs
• Exploration zone, not exercise yard
• Pet family reunions
• Free "yappie hour" with purchase of Kong toy (fill with food before feeding)
• Memorial services
• Over-40 programs for mature pets, not "geriatric exams"
• Affection connection
• Holy-mutt-ra-mony breeding programs
• People time with play time
• Doggy day care; lay like a dog as fun time
• Canine eat-sleep-play routine = stop-drop-roll
• Pet showers, pre-departure cleansing baths
• "Every Pet Deserves A Pet" awareness program
• Restoring puppy kisses, not "doing dentals"
• *Dogs, Cats, & Kids* video by Wayne Hunthausen for canine socialization
• Bayer Pet Ecosystem Management VCR

Anthropomorphic characteristics can be capitalized upon to create an awareness to get clients to listen to the needs of their pets. This concept, and these phrases, are not a gimmick; they are a communication necessity!

We Must Care

The need to convey the reason we entered veterinary medicine is critical to building that client-practice bond. No one entered practice for the short hours, the great hourly wage, or the job security. Most practitioners have an innate love of animals, a desire to alleviate suffering, and a solicitude for the people they serve when delivering concerned healthcare. But to be successful, we must convey these human–companion animal bonding traits to our clients, and they must be conveyed sincerely and consistently.

The process of thanking a client must be specific and timely to be an effective bonding technique. The first "thank you for the referral" that a client gets is just that, a tailored letter that reinforces the quality of the practice, the appreciation of the referral, and a hope that you will continue to provide the type of service that they want to refer friends to in the future. The second thank you letter says, "thank you for sending *another* client," and adds a premium as a gesture of appreciation. I have found that practice discounts are perceived as self-promotion rather than appreciation. A pair of tickets to a local movie, zoo, or animal park reflect a "no strings attached" appreciation. Some practices even send tickets to sporting events or concerts if they know it is a special interest of that client. But that means you must spend the extra moments to record these fact on the client data sheet of the medical record, and that is another issue.

Techniques That Enhance

The environment of the reception room is a mood setter. Does the practice keep *Better Homes and Gardens, People,* or *Time* magazines in the reception area so they can be bought as tax deductions, or are there client bond builders like the *Delta Society Journal, Pet Health News,* and *Latham Letter?* Does the practice keep a scrapbook in the waiting area with the pictures that have been sent by clients of your patients? Has someone taken the effort to label the scrapbook pictures with a little information about the pet, the client, and the location/situation where the picture was taken? Is there a pictorial available concerning the activities that occur in "the back room"? Our clients wonder about that mysterious place that they never go, and a collage or scrapbook or even individually framed pictures help take the mystery out and bond the client to your concern about their pet. Do the receptionist, technician, and staff address the client and patient by name at every opportunity?

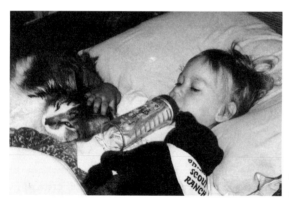

Compliments of Jessica and Meleaguer Catanzaro.

When we discuss the needs of the companion animal, does the staff address them as an advocate of the animal's well-being, or is the practice philosophy one where we try to keep a superior or professional position? Does the veterinarian tell the client what the pet "needs" for proper health maintenance or what the practice "needs" to do for comprehensive healthcare; do we allow the client to waive these services rather than make the decision for them? You'll find the pet advocate gets much more support and cooperation in the healthcare process, not to mention a larger per patient transaction fee. Does the veterinarian take time to explain the "philosophy of the practice" or does the practice cop-out with cold "clinic policies"?

Does the practice "reach out and touch someone" by mail or in person? How many follow-ups, recalls, or reminders are done by mail versus using the telephone. When following up a surgery case or an extended medication treatment plan (e.g., 21-day cystitis therapy), it isn't hard to teach the receptionist or technician to say, "Mrs. ____, this is Judi from the ____Veterinary Hospital, we know you are due back in about a week, but the doctor and I just wanted to be sure you haven't had any questions arise now that you've been home for a couple of days." When calling a new client, something like, ". . .we know you're coming back for the next puppy shots in three weeks but wanted to say we enjoyed your first visit and just wanted to be sure there aren't any new questions" can close the "doctor and I" telephone introduction.

When an appointment is missed, wouldn't it be a nice touch to show concern for the pet and client rather than the appointment log? Teach the receptionist to pick up the phone and say something like, "Mrs. Jones, this is Suzie at XYZ Veterinary Hospital, we noticed that we didn't see you as expected yesterday and the doctor and I just wanted to call and see if everything was okay at your house?" Do not continue talking after this opening statement; the first person to talk now will have to explain. Just let the client talk, and listen carefully; if clients want to reschedule, they will say so. If they are ducking an appointment, a caring, "That's fine, we just wanted to make sure your family and Fluffy were healthy and didn't need any assistance. . . . " will establish a better bond than trying to force the making of another appointment. These scripts must be practiced before they are used. The words must seem real. If you are not willing to take the time and sit together as a team to rehearse the practice narratives, then do not expect someone on staff to take the time to listen to clients.

There are many communication techniques that convey the caring and concern of a practice, but a preprinted postcard is not usually one of them. The first reminder by postcard is great, but let the practice concern show through on follow-ups. A letter or a phone call will usually achieve greater bonding results than that second postcard. A possible exception to the telephone call follow-up is in communities that are saturated with telemarketing programs that keep the family phone ringing off the hook from 6 P.M. to 8:30 P.M. In this case, the letter that appears personally written will be the best follow-up to make that client feel like a member of your practice family.

Bereavement Counseling

Times of stress require a special giving that is not taught in most veterinary schools. The stress is there with any major illness or injury and is often seen with even the most minor problem. The client is not trained to differentiate major from minor concerning a loved pet. Any client-perceived emergency or crisis is just that, and your compassion and concern starts the bereavement counseling process. The real challenge occurs in the exam room, when the stress of a pet problem makes the clients share their other life stresses with you, since grief and stress are cumulative. AAHA sells three great children's books about pet loss [*Tenth Good Thing About Barney* (Viorst), *Mister Rogers on Pet Loss,* and *I'll Always Love You* (Wilhelm)]; nonmembers can get them cheaper at any local bookstore. I have personally kept a couple of each available for loan. These books are not in lieu of caring, compassion, and concern; they are additional to those feelings shared in the exam room. The individual techniques vary with the practice, but most successful practices utilize quality time in the examination room or office and a follow-up sympathy card; many utilize donations in memory of the animal (e.g., to the Morris Animal Foundation, Cornell Feline Center, or a local wildlife park or zoo). When there are young children, I find that using a local zoo or animal park allows the parent to say, "these animals are kept well by our veterinarian in memory of Fluffy's love." A few even send a bud vase and card following a tragic experience by good clients; the technique must fit the practice's usual image and approach to caring or it will seem a hollow gesture. The bottom line is simple; it is okay to care. It is fine to feel sad, and if you cry with a client no one will think less of you.

Putting It into Action

The techniques to apply the human–companion animal bond to daily practice as discussed here are not all-inclusive, nor are techniques fail-safe methods to build a client-practice bond. The 26 appendices with practice programs *cannot* all be implemented at once; the practice leadership needs to select and implement one at a time. The sincere sharing of feelings will be accepted by the majority of our clients and, most often when exhibited appropriately and sincerely, will cause a client to keep a bond with the practice even after a pet's untimely death. Put yourself in the client's position and give the compassion that the stressful situation requires. Understand that awareness of the human–companion animal bond belongs in the practice as well as in nursing homes or other pet facilitated therapy programs.

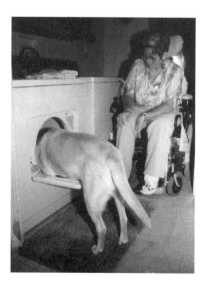

2

The Consumer's Search

HUMAN HEALTHCARE management firms have taken a closer look at how most people come to select their healthcare providers. All of the reports hold four factors as common variables: quality, relationship, convenience, and price. Each of these factors can be seen in a veterinary practice, and play an important role in bonding the client to the practice.

Trade-Offs

The average consumer today wants options. Price is obviously only one element in the purchasing process. It has been found to be critical only when the healthcare consumer does not have a strong preference for a hospital. If the quality of two providers is perceived as similar, consumers will then match price against other attributes to determine which combination provides the most value.

Based on market research of potential healthcare consumers, price was ranked tenth in importance among 14 variables. Instead of price, they look at factors such as doctors, support staff, facilities, courtesy, convenience, modern equipment, services, and other physical indicators. While most consumers don't see paying less as a trade-off for quality or amenities, they do have a price range in mind. In the veterinary community, the numbers are similar to those in human healthcare. Veterinary client research (Anderson et al. 1984) has shown that $250 to $300 is the current decision point for about half the clients; up to that point, "Do what you need to do to fix our pet" is usually a true statement. After that point, discretionary spending pressures come into the equation to offset the values associated with the human-animal bond.

Today's client makes assumptions about both hospital price and hospital quality. The human healthcare researchers revealed that consumers believe that quality varies between hospitals. They have also found that most clients generally relate higher price to better care.

Perceptions of Price vs. Quality

The research on the clients' perceptions of price in human healthcare are intriguing:

- Only 17 percent ever believed they had a low-priced hospital; the majority view their hospital prices as the same or more than other hospitals in the area.
- One-fourth report that hospitals with low prices lead them to believe that they are also of lower quality.
- Three out of 10 believe if they pay more they will receive higher quality care.
- Over half of consumers are willing to pay higher prices to receive care from a hospital they view as offering the highest quality healthcare.
- Four out of 10 healthcare consumers report they would prefer a hospital with an image of good quality and low price to a hospital with an image of high quality and high price. They also don't feel technical quality is an issue among these hospitals.

Past Experience

Consumers without relationships with a healthcare provider or facility are more likely to look at price differences simply because other trade-off variables are not known. This is a characteristic of human nature; decisions are made based on the knowledge at hand. Remember the old adage, "When people don't know what to do, they do what they know"? This applies to human healthcare as well as veterinary practice selection, pet dietary programs, animal dental hygiene, and a host of other informational factors that we are supposed to share with clients on a regular basis.

Past experience moved your practice to where it is today, but it won't get you into tomorrow. Leadership and vision are required in the 2000s. In the case of consumer targeted marketing, leadership is being comfortable with being out of control; the team should be able to carry the practice dream effectively into tomorrow.

One-third of healthcare consumers who have a regular provider say they would switch if they could find one who was of equal or better quality but less expensive. A slightly smaller group was willing to switch for better hours or a closer location if quality would not decrease. A third group would switch because of inconvenience and the extra time involved in waiting for an appointment.

Shaping Strategy

As you develop pricing strategies, make sure you evaluate the practice's market segment based on the value your clients place on these factors:

- Quality of services
- Loyalty to practice and staff
- Location/convenience
- Fair fee schedule

Using these factors and a client segment profile, you can position your veterinary practice as a high quality but reasonably priced provider of pet healthcare, a low-price provider with equitable quality, or a number of other options. No matter what tactic you choose, the scenario hinges on the ability of your clients to make informed choices. Unfortunately, it is often clear that veterinary clients do not have the necessary information to compare provider prices and performance.

It is critical that we use our communication skills to increase the client's veterinary IQ while we try to bond the client to the practice. When we have helped our clients understand the factors that go into quality care and fair fees, misrepresentations by others will become glaringly clear. As the client's veterinary IQ increases, it is essential to respond to the client with better information and a clearer set of options in pet healthcare.

Increasing client veterinary IQ will also make it important for our staff to develop effective communication skills. The future is ours to harvest, so we need to develop our training efforts now to meet the needs of tomorrow. If we believe that our market niche lies in well-informed veterinary consumers, consumer perceptions become an important factor to manage for our practice image. Quality is relative, as are perceptions, and both can be managed by a caring veterinary healthcare delivery team.

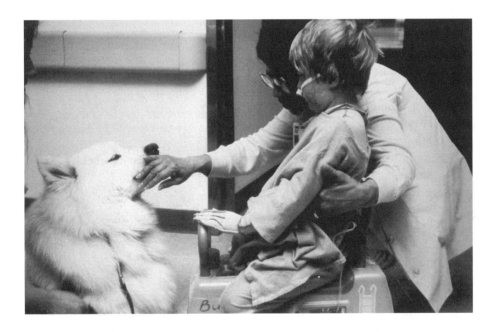

Veterinary Practice Images

He who knows much about others may be learned, but he who knows himself is more intelligent. He who controls others may be more powerful, but he who has mastered himself is mightier still.

—Lao Tsu

Image. We talk about a practice image, a professional image, an image of caring. What are you doing, on a daily basis, to improve that image? In the current management literature, a new buzz phrase has emerged: "moments of truth." It was coined by the CEO of Scandinavian Airlines System (Jan Carlzon) and means simply "an opportunity to influence a customer, to create an appropriate image." In every encounter with every person, at least one moment of truth occurs. Generally, more than a single moment occurs in each encounter to make an impression. In each instance, impressions and values are established based on impressions and perceptions. In a veterinary practice, these moments of truth are often the difference between a client becoming a four-times-per-year friend or a once-in-three-years visitor.

In a brainstorming session with other consultants, we looked at the average veterinary practice client cycle and counted the moments of truth that any practice could possibly influence. While all the ideas listed here will not fit every practice, the majority should. The challenge is to get the staff members to accept the responsibility for improving the image in each area they touch. They need to have pride in what they do, moment by moment, to affect these moments of truth. To establish that pride in performance is the challenge of leadership, but that is a different book! Look at the following opportunities and discuss them with your team:

Finding the practice
    Yellow page ad
    Referral by client
    Newspaper ad
    Community literature source
    Referral by out-of-state veterinarian
    Outdoor signage
Ancillary pet supply referral
    Staff community service
    Community activities/Rotary/Scouting/women's clubs/government
The initial contact
    Phone for a price quote
    Phone for a service quote
    Phone for an appointment
    Directions to the practice
    Stopping in for a tour
    Meeting a staff member out in the community
    Meeting the veterinarian at a community function
    Actual appointment hours offered
Arriving with the pet
    Practice identification
    Direction signage for parking and entrance
    Parking lot appearance/tidiness/potholes/debris/droppings
    Access to the front door
    Entry ease and protection of pet from other patients
    Lighting/security
    Initial waiting room impression
    Access to the front desk
    Staff appearance
    Decor/odor/noise/cleanliness

Reception staff
   Courtesy/attentiveness
   Friendliness/smiles
   Responsiveness/caring
   Pace/professional approach
   Phone techniques
Gossip level
   Talk about pets/clients by name rather than condition
   Waiting time
   Amenities available
   Other clients entering and exiting (satisfaction)
Initial client/patient movement methods
   Appearance/uniforms/shoes/personal composure
   Personal hygiene/makeup/hair/breath/facial hair
   Escort to examination room
   Initial interview techniques
   Hands on pet within 30 seconds
   Technician appearance
   Body language/voice tone
   Staff competency
   Paraprofessional rapport
   Wellness examination
   Diplomas on wall
   Odor/cleanliness/noise
Veterinarian initial impact
   Appearance/personal composure
   Treatment of staff
   Self-introduction
   Touching the animal
   Listening technique
   Body language/voice tone/rate of speech
   Terminology
   Explanation of examination/findings
   Patient advocacy/speaks of pet's needs/ensures client decides
   Empathy/concern for client's position (emotional and fiscal)
Examination Room Exit
   Summary of findings
   Training to administer treatments
   Explanation of charges
   Prequalify each departure with the three Rs (recheck, recall, reminders)
   Escort to discharge
   Protection of animal during transit through hall/reception area
Discharge actions
   Attentiveness at discharge/waiting time
   Discharge desk clutter/appearance

Cleanliness/odor/noise
Presentation of invoice/bill (consistency with estimate)
Collection of fees
Dispensing medication
Concern for client understanding
Establishing three Rs compliance expectations/methodology
Privacy/courtesy/caring
Literature offered to ensure family understanding
Postdischarge actions
Follow-up telephone call/newsletters
Sympathy cards/memorials for deceased pets
"Thank you" correspondence
Satisfaction surveys
Reminders

Over 100 moments of truth were listed above, and the ability of the veterinarian to directly alter them accounted for only about 10 percent of the total. The amount of concern (training and rehearsal) exhibited by most veterinary practices does not equal the importance of these client impression opportunities.

Consider the moments of truth from the client's perspective. How many times can your staff, facility, or practice methods negatively impress a client before he/she is no longer a client? Conversely, every moment of truth is an opportunity to cement the doctor-client-patient bond.

In fact, as has been proven in most every service industry, how operational managers and supervisors treat staff will determine how staff members treat clients. When Carlzon asked the Scandinavian Airlines System (SAS) headquarters staff what their mission was, it took three weeks for the team to decide it was "the movement of people." They closed the headquarters for about six months and took the client-centered service to the field to impress every one of the 40,000 employees with their importance in the moments of truth. In two years, SAS went from a failing airline to one of the top three income producers in Europe. But they rested on their 1988–89 performance and forgot to reinforce the client-centered programs. They forgot to look into the future and make the SAS employees responsible for change in the future. SAS lost money.

The successful practice empowers its staff to react and change to meet the clients' needs: to be free to commit resources without additional line item permission and to make the client perceive a caring staff and a quality healthcare facility. In human healthcare this concept is called continuous quality improvement (CQI). In industry and corporate America it has been called total quality management (TQM). Authors like Juran, Deming, and Crosby have made their consulting fame by reintroducing employee-based quality and pride factors to American corporations. They believe that when employees put pride into their daily effort, when they are empowered to make changes for the betterment of the team without first climbing the supervisory ladder for permission, the output will be perceived as quality.

Accountability assigned to an employee (empowerment) must be accompanied by the needed authority, and these must be supported by job/task ownership. The staff member must think of the practice as "our practice/our hospital" at every decision point in the process. In the consulting business, we find that practice "luck" is usually directly related to the preparation of the staff to grab opportunity as it comes knocking. Where does your practice approach sit in the scheme of things when it comes to preparing your staff to grab the moment of truth and turn it to the practice's advantage?

The trend in the United States during the past few decades has been away from client service. However, the 1990s have rediscovered the importance of service to the client. American examples such as Marriott, Nordstrom, Worthington Steel, Federal Express, and American Airlines do exist, but they are the exception rather than the rule. 2000 must bring an increase in client service!

The practice that best controls its respective moments of truth will become different from other practices in the minds of the community. These astute veterinary practices will succeed where others have floundered because practice quality and client impressions are communicated during the moments of truth and have very little bearing on the professional facts. They will become the leaders in the veterinary marketplace during this decade.

The First Impression: What Does the Client See?

In American veterinary practice, we can't accept congestion; we must combat the first impression that is accepted by the community. When people bring their animals to the veterinarian, they are often stressed. If they are also worrying about the proximity of a near-by animal and the danger it presents to their pet, the stress is compounded. Clients are worried about their animal's health, and they are worried about the size of the bill when the doctor is done. A stressed person needs reinforcement for their decision to access your practice as well as for the "correctness" of their decisions after the examination.

When the client selects your practice, a first impression is formed, especially if it was due to a positive word-of-mouth referral. They will be expecting a similar level of service and care. When they look for a parking space, what will they find? Is your practice clearly marked, or does a client have to know how to find you before the small name plate by the door is evident? Does the building look dilapidated or dirty, with poorly kept lawn, weed-ridden flower beds, fecal deposits, or other "negative wellness" signals? Clients often perceive veterinary healthcare in terms of the outward appearances, including weak or dead plants in the reception area.

Other reception area detractors are smell, sight, and sound; hopefully these are well controlled within your practice. In some practices, keeping these sensations from "floating forward" requires a consistent reminder to the staff; in others, automatic door closers have solved the problem without the constant lectures by the boss. The reception area should have recent, animal friendly reading material; pictures should be framed; and there should be a quality selection of brochures and handouts from which the client can select items to take home and read later.

The floors in a practice are a constant problem, and some practices have hired a janitorial service to clean them during a slow mid-week, mid-day time, rather than always yelling at the staff. The staff still needs to be aware of cleanliness, especially urine accidents or blood drips that need immediate cleaning; the mop bucket needs to be close to the front and ready to use at all times. Make it easy for staff to keep the front client areas clean and shiny.

When the practice slows down during the winter months, the staff also seems to slow down. The practice deteriorates. This is the time to do maintenance chores. Who keeps the list in your practice, how can people add things, and how are items prioritized for action? When was the last time the corners got a new coat of paint to cover the leash rubs; when were the examination room wall dividers, curtains, or wallpaper changed? When were the ceiling light covers cleaned last or the cobwebs in the ceiling corners removed? Looking up as well as down is important! If the colors or decor have not been changing every five years or so, the client perception is often that "old and out-of-date" care is provided at the facility.

If we believe Jan Carlzon of the Scandinavian Airlines System (SAS), the client experience is a series of small episodes; each is a "moment of truth" to be managed or ignored. As a practice manages individual moments of truth, it also influences client perceptions and loyalty. Moments of truth can be nurtured, and a positive experience occurs; or they can be overlooked, and a negative impression is carried away. Clients with a positive first experience will probably return and be more likely to accept the services offered for their animals. Managing the first impression means taking the time to train the staff to address all the small things, over 100 by my last count, that a client encounters in the veterinary examination visit.

You can't do it by yourself; it is a team effort. The veterinary healthcare delivery team includes everyone who comes in contact with the animal, the client, or the facility; each has a way of influencing the client. The even coat of paint on the door trim, the smell of the pet's coat when it leaves your back room, and the tone of the voice answering the phone for the practice are each a moment of truth that requires attention and recurring management emphasis. The client's perception of the difference between practices is usually based on neither professional skill nor cost of equipment, but rather on the practice team's effort toward managing the client encounter and exceeding the individual client's expectation(s).

The veterinary practice staff needs to continually assess the patient's experience through the eyes and feelings of the client. They need to be trusted to make changes, additions, and deletions to procedures that further stress or alienate a client. They need to be asked to continuously improve their client service as well as their client image efforts. The pride the staff shows in meeting the client's expectations will generally be perceived as quality by the clients. Meeting this need and conveying this image may be the *only difference needed* to make your practice special in your community.

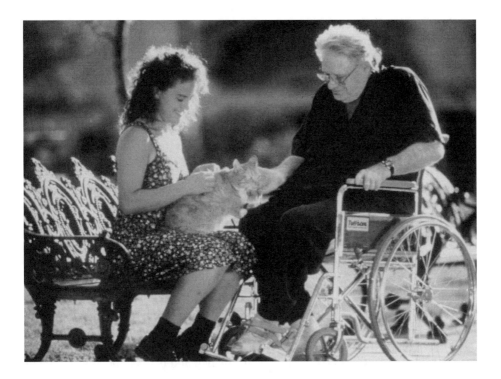

Courtesy, a Client Contact Must

*Always let your client keep their dignity, then appeal to their
sense of doing what is fair and right.*
—Dr. T.E. Catanzaro

Recently, I stood in line at an airport in the northeast and learned firsthand how not to treat a client. When I reached the front of the airline's roped off "cattle chute" system for passengers waiting to see a ticket agent, which had already been a 30-minute ordeal, the agent reached up and pulled down a sign reading, "This line is closed." Without a word of apology or explanation, she went on her "break" (an assumption by a fellow sufferer who was a bit more vocal than I). I was infuriated also but had just made a mental note to change my travel profile with my agent so I will *never* access that airline again. I don't begrudge any staff member the needed break, but in any service industry, whether it be airline, veterinary medicine, or retail sales, courtesy is critical at all times.

How often have you had a similar experience—perhaps in a bank, in a restaurant, or with a supplier? How did you feel after the encounter? How often do you review the telephone techniques of the staff, the receptionist script on what is expected by clients, or other "rules" developed for clients? Why do we develop rules for clients rather than options? Is it a logic sequence gone astray, or is it a bad habit we learned in the past whose impact on our own clients we have never assessed? The main lesson is this: *Persons in contact with the public must be courteous all the time!*

Courtesy has been called many things—hospitality, tact, pleasantness, politeness, good cheer, thoughtfulness, charm, smile training, or like mom used to say, just a good set of "company manners." Simply put, courtesy means being nice to people—being the kind of person who gets along with everyone. Being nice often means listening to their frustrations, their worries, or their concerns. In business, courtesy is a must!

But let's face it, being courteous is not always easy, especially for receptionists. There are times when being courteous can be a pain in the neck; these are the days when being courteous can ruin your day. For example:

- When you take a late-afternoon phone call from a well-known chronic complainer. She is a good client and has many pets, but always seems to call at the discharge rush hour with petty complaints. No matter what has been done, there seems to be a problem with each practice encounter.
- You are face-to-face with a client who thinks they know a lot more about veterinary medical advances than the doctor or staff of your practice. This client may suggest impossible procedures or expensive diagnostics they want for free, ask irrelevant questions, or make unreasonable demands of your time or the resources of the practice.
- And then there are the times you are required to calm the angry client. Despite your best efforts, this person remains unsatisfied and is likely becoming downright rude.

It is impossible to avoid such experiences. Every practice has them. They are part of each practice day. The majority of them can be defused with simple questions, such as, "What can we do to make it right for you?" or a simple statement such as, "That is an interesting viewpoint I hadn't considered; let me pass that on to the doctor and have him/her call you later." Not everyone has a doctor who can tactfully defuse a situation, but there should be staff members skilled in client negotiations who are authorized to "make it right."

Clients also respond to "pedestal words," those brief words or phrases that raise the client to a level above the ordinary. It is a real plus in courtesy training when the team learns to make clients feel they have been put onto a pedestal. Here are 10 examples to try as a starting point:

- *May I?* (Asking permission implies authority.)
- *As you of course know* . . . (Implies vast knowledge.)
- *I'd like your advice.* (Suggests superior wisdom.)
- *I'd sure appreciate it if* . . . (There is an implication here that the client has the power to refuse or grant a favor.)
- *You are so right.* (A pat on the back.)
- *. . . spare time from your busy life* . . . (Implies the client is a busy and therefore important person.)
- *Because of your knowledge* . . . (Implies an understanding and professional skill.)
- *. . . a person of your standing* . . . (No one knows just what standing means but everyone believes—or hopes—he/she has it.)

• *I'd like your considered opinion.* (Clients on pedestals are supposed to have opinions, so if an opinion is asked, the client must be up there somewhere, and becomes part of the solution.)
• *Please.* (A great lubricator in human relations.)

Whether you use a caring approach, pedestal words, or a combination of techniques, your popularity will grow. You achieve a real victory when you deal with unhappy clients or disagreeable situations in a positive way, by being pleasantly and efficiently courteous. It is a victory that makes everyone a winner—the practice, the staff, and the client. Courtesy is an absolute essential in every client contact. You can never let down your guard. The practice, and the clients, are depending on you.

Focusing on the Client

Clients should be first, staff second, owners third, and communities fourth, so says Robert Waterman who with Tom Peters authored the 1981 management bible *In Search of Excellence*. It has been over a decade since the research for this book was done, but most of the principles remain valid today. Organizations that stay close to their consumers stay focused on what is important.

The Shrinking Caddy

In 1984, General Motors (GM) listened to their engineers and Congress, then shrank the Cadillac by two feet. Sales stalled, forcing GM to rethink their car design program. They met with five groups of Caddy owners, 500 owners per group, over a three-year period. They put these people behind the wheel of prototypes and let them play. The result was the 1988 Cadillac DeVille and Fleetwood that cruised into showrooms with subtle tail fins, nine extra inches, fender skirts, and a 36 percent sales growth over a year earlier. The Caddy "gunboat" was back, and overall volume had grown for the first time in five years.

A tough lesson was driven home: pay great attention to the consumer and know their real desires. Forum Corporation, a Boston-based consulting firm that specializes in consumer service, has shown that keeping a customer typically costs only one-fifth as much as acquiring a new one.

Staying Close

As veterinarians, we have learned what is best for the animal. We care, but often we do not listen. I have spoken often of patient advocacy, the concept of speaking to the client on behalf of the pet's welfare. This carries with it the obligation to listen to the replies. We must think of ourselves as the client if we want to communicate.

The art of communication, and staying close to the client, is an art of caring. There are a few basic rules to follow to make it happen.

• Always remember that our clients are not dependent on us—we are dependent on them. They are the important people in any practice.

- Respond quickly and directly. Answer their question first. Be ready to acknowledge perceived bad service did occur.
- Match their rate of speech in a language they understand. Ensure your body language and voice tone match the message you are stating.
- Make every staff member aware of your practice dream and ensure everyone sends the same message.
- Monitor service internally to see that your staff treat one another like you want clients treated. You can't afford to have a bad day.
- Listen to everyone in your client contact chain and respect internal thinking. You can't respond until you know the perceived message.
- Reduce the barrier of professional detachment so clients feel free to talk to you. Learn to act rather than react.
- Stay in touch after the healthcare episode. Caring should not stop with the "cure."

Checks and Balances

Northwestern Mutual Insurance relies on their clients to "calibrate" the company headquarters annually. Since 1907, five policy owners, recommended by field agents, are brought in annually to be demanding, no-nonsense parents and tell the staff what it is they are doing right and wrong. They spend five days interviewing officers, examining documents, snooping for problems, and watching the bureaucracy. Nothing and no one is off limits. The company prints the group's review unedited in its annual report. Would you be willing to put your practice up to that level of review? If you see your clients as you, it should be a welcomed service.

Northwestern Mutual has a 95 percent renewal rate, the industry's highest retention rate. One of the key reasons is the annual on-site review by the policy holder group. Tom Moraghan of Domino's Pizza has been getting close to his customers by paying 10,000 families to be "mystery customers." Each family agrees to buy 23 pizzas from Domino's throughout the year to evaluate quality and service. A manager's bonus compensation is partly based on those scores. The regional offices rate the corporate Domino's staff monthly on the quality of service they receive, and the monthly bonuses paid to every full-time home office worker are based in part on the evaluations.

Some veterinary practices use client surveys (sample follows) and become discouraged by the unremarkable replies. This is due in part to the sample group. Our clients like us and don't want to hurt our feelings. They "understand" our long hours and harried appearance. They know mistakes happen and forgive us our errors without our having to ask. But what of our new clients or the clients picking up their records because they are leaving? If we really cared, we would interview these two populations of clients for their opinions. Review the list of potential target questions below to develop ideas for your own practice. We need to believe what these clients tell us since perceptions are "fact" for those that hold them.

SAMPLE NEW CLIENT QUESTIONS:
Did we discuss all the pets in your household?   Y   N
Are you adequately informed of the Lyme Disease threat in _____? Y   N

Were you informed that we have a modern cat boarding facility?   Y   N
Are you aware of the heartworm danger to dogs in this community?   Y   N
Did we discuss the wellness healthcare needs of cats   Y   N
in this community?
Did we offer the level of quality care you expected for your pet?   Y   N
Were you allowed to waive or defer care that you did not wish given?   Y   N
Were you given our emergency telephone number for 24-hour care?   Y   N
Do you know this hospital offers nutritional counseling for pets?   Y   N
Did we tell you about our parasite prevention and control counseling?   Y   N
Is your pet on a routine dental hygiene program?   Y   N

How did you FIRST hear about our practice:
___ Friend (who may we thank?_____)
___ Signage by the practice
___ Yellow pages because of location
___ Yellow pages because of services published
___ Referral because of AAHA status
___ Specialty referral by another veterinarian or pet shop
___ Other_____

DEPARTING CLIENT QUESTIONS:
    What one thing/service/person encountered at this hospital was important enough to you that you'll look for it at your next veterinarian's practice?

_____
_____
_____

    What one thing did you encounter at this practice that you never want to experience again?

_____
_____
_____

    Please prioritize the reasons you initially selected this practice, then list your current reason(s) for leaving (1 most, 5 least concern):

Initial Selection Priority	Reason	Exit Priority
_____	Location of practice	_____
_____	Friend's recommendation	_____
_____	Yellow page promises	_____
_____	Pet shop recommendation	_____
_____	Signage/appearance	_____
_____	Inexpensive prices	_____
_____	Quality care	_____
_____	Staff courtesy	_____
_____	Veterinarian's ability	_____

Initial Selection Priority	Reason	Exit Priority
_____	Family atmosphere	_____
_____	Understandable doctor	_____
_____	Concerned healthcare	_____

The alternative to the written client survey is the "council of clients" approach. This group is comprised of those who paid the most in the previous quarter. You need at least 8 households represented, preferably 10, at an after-dinner dessert function. The reason: to improve the community support for this practice. There only need to be two or three attendees from the practice: let the clients out number the team. Ask questions and wear a very thick skin! There is no defense against perceptions, so do not offer justifications at this "council of clients" survey time. You can ask for their opinion on how to convey the information. For example, with dentals:

Client: The dental prices are too high, they are twice what I pay for my kids!
Practice: You are right. Children do not require anesthesia but pets do, for their safety as well as ours. For an anesthetic patient, we must do pre-anesthetic laboratory screens and physical examinations, and we have postanesthetic recovery concerns. What would be the best way to let clients know of the care we provide in the process of a dental procedure?

The "council of clients" is an indicator, not the final word. If the same problem comes up two quarters in a row, it should be addressed quickly. Actions stemming from the council-of-clients input should be published in some form so they and your other clients can see what you are doing to better serve the community. The concept of asking a client how your practice is doing is very scary, but it has worked for many industries. They are the purchasers of your services. This way, you can really meet their needs, especially if you ask, "What else should we be offering you as a pet owner or us as a healthcare facility?"

In the short run, client perceptions can harm the ego, but in the long run they can improve the practice. A practice that responds to the client will grow and develop as a service to the community. A practice that makes excuses and "explains away" the perceptions of the clients is doomed to stagnation. The choice in the next decade is yours. Bloom or stagnate. You decide which end of the olfactory spectrum you would like to be on.

References

Anderson, R.K., B.L. Hart, and L.A. Hart (eds.). 1984. *The Pet Connection: Its Influence on Our Health and Quality of Life.* Minneapolis: Center to Study Human-Animal Relationships and Environments (CENSHARE), University of Minnesota.

The Obligation to Serve

Glory is fleeting, but obscurity is forever.
—Napoleon Bonaparte

TODAY'S HEALTHCARE market allows the selective patient to choose his/her hospital, and the density of quality healthcare facilities in our urban areas allows virtually all patients to choose their hospitals for second encounters. The effective healthcare managers are constantly alert for actions or programs that give the perception of more or improved services as well as those activities that may cause dissatisfaction among their patients or the patients' families. While the proposed national healthcare programs appear to want to curtail these advantages, the rules are still valid today. These statements of fact apply to human healthcare and veterinary healthcare equally.

Pets in Healthcare—In-Roads to Success

The strength of the human-animal bond has been well documented by publications of the Delta Society and its conferences and meetings. The role of animals in reducing stress and anxiety has been well accepted by healthcare providers, although the mechanisms are still debatable. The publications of CENSHARE at the University of Minnesota, *The Pet Connection,* and subsequent periodicals laid to rest the early concerns of disease and damage that had been predicted by those fearful of animals in healthcare facilities. For instance, in 12 months in 284 facilities in Minnesota, no disease was transmitted and only 19 minor mechanical injuries had occurred (scratches, chicken peck, tripped over leash, etc.). Even the injuries due to leash errors were in violation of the protocols that precluded patients from walking pets.

These same studies have alluded to better patient harmony and an improved staff attitude when animals are involved if the involvement was voluntary. In any apprehensive healthcare delivery situation, such as pediatric oncology, hospice, or geriatric nursing, forced involvement from healthcare providers causes negative responses. When clinical expertise and animal interest are both present, however, patient care time often decreases due to the pets' fulfilling the patient's need for caring interaction. Programs have been tailored to fit the facilities' needs and restrictions vary from pet visitation programs to a central facility location, to bedside visitation programs, to the in-room bonding program. While in-room boarding of patient pets increase private room marketing success, human–companion animal bond programs have a far greater impact.

The mental anguish of a pet owner separated from his/her animals is significant. Most research has shown that three out of four pet owners believe that their pets are members of their families. Seventy-five percent is a significant proportion when we understand that over half of our population are pet owners. The stewardship felt by pet owners extends to the care and feeding of their "wards," especially during acute care episodes when preplanning has not occurred. Concern for out-of-facility pet care for inpatients, with or without visitation programs, gives the perception of increased concerned care. This may be no more than a couple of simple questions on all admission forms to query on pet ownership and interim pet care provisions.

When a pet and owner are reunited after a protracted hospital stay, the tears of joy tell the significance of the bond. As we encounter the oncology ward that has walled contact out, whether due to death or sensory overload, we see the introduction of animals as a means of opening the doors and windows to life. The non-judgmental love of a ward mascot is often the difference between satisfying and dissatisfying working environments for staff members as well as patients.

In today's healthcare delivery spectrum, increased competition causes the constant need to increase a facility's patient market share. The competitive edge goes to the facility that meets the community's needs while minimizing additional costs in material or manpower resources. Contemporary pet programs like active pet selection assistance, pets by prescription, and behavior management do just that while supporting the healthcare reverence for life and quality of care programs.

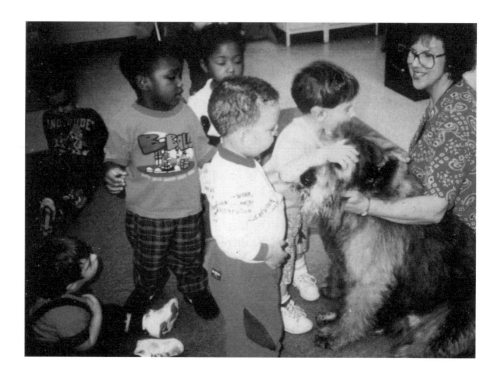

Establishing the Psychological Bond

Pet Selection

The American Veterinary Medical Association has developed and makes available all the documents and aids needed for active pet selection assistance by veterinary practices, including very well done color brochures. The Delta Society has developed the protocols for pets by prescription within the community and school environment. Either of these programs develop new pet owners, clients who are already bonded to the practice since they selected their pet with the expert assistance of the veterinary professionals of the practice.

Behavior Management

Behavior management is another potential practice area, and the head collar by Ameri-Pet, Inc., has allowed behavior changes to be facilitated in minutes rather than weeks, as previously encountered in "obedience training" sessions. Behavior management has also emerged in Japan, with Ms. Terry Ryan conducting multiple programs every year. Regardless of the country, the state, or the city, most animals lose their homes, and often their lives, because of behavior problems. The practice which helps prevent this "disposable pet" syndrome not only keeps clients, but gains recognition in the community. Recognition for helping animals is a marketing benefit to the practice, gained without having to advertise or market routine services or products.

Human–Companion Animal Bond (H-CAB) Programs

Resources are available at almost no cost to the veterinary healthcare facility. There are multiple human–companion animal bond (H-CAB) programs available from nonprofit organizations. The international clearing house for interdisciplinary H-CAB groups and programs is the Delta Society (206/226-7357). The American Veterinary Medical Association (708/925-8070) has pet placement information. Use of these groups has to be controlled and monitored to ensure they meet proper healthcare guidelines. Any good program will include at least the following six basic techniques with documented implementation planning:

1. Screening of staff and patients for bias or acceptance toward H-CAB programs.
2. Screening and quarantine procedures for any animal used in the program.
3. Volunteer training and indoctrination program before their participation.
4. Health records and preventive medicine parameters for participating animals.
5. Continuing education and in-service training at recurring intervals for facility staff due to employment turnover.
6. Evaluation of program benefits and problems for patients and staff.

As an evaluation process, the astute healthcare administrator challenges the animal facilitated therapy programs with an open mind, but with a jaundiced eye toward longevity. The people who facilitate the program must be ready to participate for the long term and should have nonprofit backing to allow the program to develop. Once the H-CAB program has proven to be effective, it should become a budget line item of the facility to ensure continuity and control.

H-CAB Benefit Inventory

The progressive veterinary practice understands that client bonding is the secret to success in an overcrowded veterinary community, and marketing of its patient advocacy philosophy feeds this image. Active participation in human-animal bond programs is usually good for free press, often to including television and radio.

A secondary benefit that results is the sensitivity of the practice staff to the emotions involved in the human–companion animal bond, which in turn softens the harshness seen in some client relations. It is also a great ego boost for support staff members when they get accolades and the "warm fuzzies" associated with an outreach program involving animals. It is the best recognition program available for many veterinary practice staff members.

The windfall benefits take many forms, sometimes including a great increase in white collar clients (doctors, teachers, healthcare professionals) who have come into contact with the human–companion animal programs that your staff supports. The client who has a full realization of the human–companion animal importance will be more likely to do what is needed for proper healthcare maintenance of the family animal(s). They take their stewardship seriously.

The only difference between being a special practice and an average practice is the desire to do a little extra to be perceived as unique in your community. The choice is yours. Capitalize on the original covenant as the provider of animal welfare and wellness. Care enough to become committed. Dare to become more than average.

Pet Population Dynamics: Why Are There Too Many Euthanasias?

I remember when I returned from an interdisciplinary pet overpopulation workshop at the University of Minnesota. Everyone with a national interest was represented, from the American Humane Association, the Humane Society of the United States, the American Society for the Prevention of Cruelty to Animals, the American Kennel Club, and Cat Fanciers, to the American Veterinary Medical Association and the American Animal Hospital Association. The meeting was also loaded with academic researchers, epidemiologists, population scientists, and others who care about too many animals being killed every year.

Two Decades of Inertia

The main impact of the workshop on me was the amazing fact that the problem has not changed after 20 years of these types of meetings. Granted, strays have decreased in cities were there are strict leash laws. Veterinarians have experienced this decrease with the low number of "hit by car" patients they are seeing. We are still killing between 5 and 25 million animals a year because they do not have homes. Some of these have to be euthanized, due to their feral nature, nonsocial behavior, or medical indications, but not millions. Like an iceberg in a shipping lane, the problem has been seen but not completely defined. Some have looked at the tip of the iceberg, others have tried to assess the size of the entire iceberg, but no one has researched the cause of the iceberg.

As a management diagnostician, not an academic researcher, I was asked to be an information resource for the meeting. The first big definition hurdle was to get a handle on "pet overpopulation." There was great discussion, but the consensus settled on the simple statement that "too many animals were being euthanized each year." Then we had to define "too many," so we came up with a simple formula:

$$\frac{\text{births } (- \text{ medically indicated euthanasias}) - \text{natural deaths}}{\text{number of responsible pet owners } (\times \text{ multi-pets})} = 1$$

Then we started looking at the factors impacting on each element of the formula, and looked at any assumptions we were making that could not be measured. In fact, none of the elements had ever been actually measured with any statistical accuracy. So we looked at clear definitions. The definition of responsible pet owner was one such challenge in clarity. We have never researched the "profile" of a responsible pet owner, or for that matter, an irresponsible pet owner. The Delta Society had a lot of data on the human-animal bond, but this question appeared too subjective for research grant funding (isn't that why we do research?). So we defined irresponsible pet owners as a percentage of the animal-owning public:

$$(1- \text{ percentage responsible pet owners}) \times 100 = \text{irresponsible percent}$$

To the researcher, this made sense; to practitioners it is still "fuzzy math." As a consultant, I count "responsible pet owners" as those who see their veterinarian annually *and* keep their animal protected from the diseases of the community.

This great exercise in pursuit of a better definition did bring us closer to the real challenge that has caused these decades of inertia. Why haven't the humane groups, local community leaders, or veterinary medical groups been able to solve this problem? In the 1980s, the mayors of the United States placed stray (uncontrolled) animals in the top three problems of urban America. Caring people have been addressing the pet overpopulation "assumption" from their own perspective. Do we have too many pets or too few responsible owners; do we see too many births or not enough natural deaths; or is it a population dynamics factor that is not easily defined?

With the guidance of Drs. Glickman and Patronek, pathobiology researchers from Purdue University, we attempted to develop a model of population dynamics as they appear today, with the basic assumption that this dynamic population (animal or human) constantly seeks a form of equilibrium (supply and demand).

This model is noteworthy because of the relationships (arrows); we don't know the values (impact) of the various elements. If there were good research,

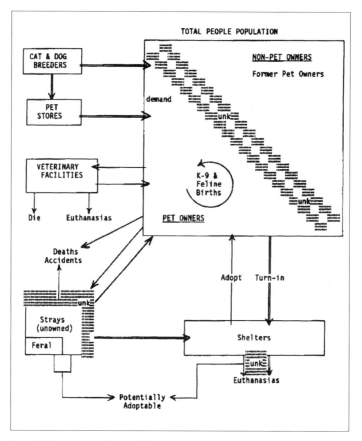

Population dynamic model

we would know the intensities of demand within a population (perhaps a county). When one population is defined, then the second population could be surveyed and compared, with the variances being validated for "cause and effect" relationships. If we look at current efforts, such as licensure, where does that impact this model? Is taxation a method of controlling pet reproduction, or is registration needed for returning lost pets? With this model, anyone can see that these issues become very small contributors to the success or failure of any community problem.

If we look at the dynamics with the "pet-owning" segment of the total population, additional relationships become very evident.

Pet Dynamics

Even with these two models for pet and human dynamics, we don't know the values or intensities that influence the equilibrium. If we compare Europe with the United States, the stray animal problems are different. Why would this be? Why are breed types, ears and tails included, different between the two populations? Why are animals more acceptable in public places in Europe? Which values are different: the animal's reproductive urges, the community mores, the animal owners themselves, or . . .? How could a similar set of values be economically introduced into an American population? Would the values cause the same results? How would we measure the changes?

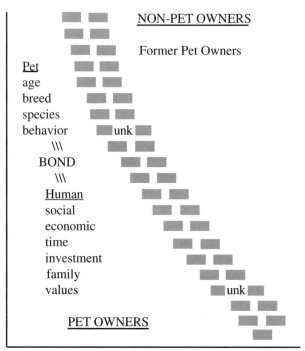

HUMAN DYNAMICS

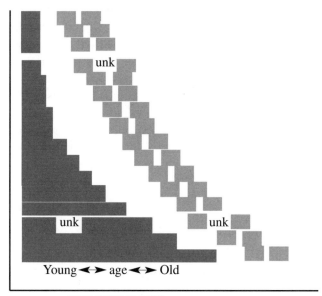

PET DYNAMICS

Human and pet dynamics.

For 20 years we have been picking at this problem from the edge but have never addressed the total causative parameters. Only an interdisciplinary effort can ever hope to address the causes and effects which require millions of animals to be killed annually at shelters and veterinary facilities across the nation.

The Alternatives

Remember, I am a management diagnostician, not a researcher. I look at what could be done, today, with very little expense, to start getting a handle on the problem. There are about 3500 shelters in the United States (no one knows for sure how many). There are about 17,400 companion animal exclusive veterinary practices (no one knows for sure). If the powers in both movements (e.g., ASPCA, AHA, HSUS, AVMA, AAHA, etc.) got together and developed a single "values survey" for pet owners, a statistically valid sample could be obtained from a portion of the existing facilities with existing staff resources. This could be compared to existing Delta Society research for human-animal bond relationships,

Are there behavior management courses that could be offered within a community, shelter, or veterinary practice which would stem the euthanasia impulse? Most people do perceive behavior problems in their pets, and responsible pet owners either accept the animal's ways or try to get professional assistance in the resolution of the behavior problem. Irresponsible pet owners ignore the animal's ways or dispose of the animal (release, turn-in, euthanasia, etc.). The current research shows about 85 percent of the behavior problems are manageable without putting the owner through prolonged obedience training.

A more expensive alternative is the "total county profile." There are methods to statistically survey a population by telephone (but you miss the non-phone households, a statistically important population in some areas of the country). New Zealand has developed a protocol for surveying stray animal populations which could likely be adapted to the United States. Non–pet owners must be profiled to determine if there is a factor that could be used to increase the number of available households (we are aware that housing restrictions are artificially limiting the pet-owning population potentials).

If we don't address this dynamic situation from an interdisciplinary viewpoint, if we don't "release our turf" and share, I don't see any great opportunity for resolution of this situation. No one can do it alone, we have proven that in the past two decades. If we don't change, we will continue to kill too many animals every year.

Why Do Clients Come?

If you build it, they will come.
    —from *Field of Dreams*

In the movie *Field of Dreams, "If you build it, they will come"* was spoken by a voice, then a corn field was plowed under, a ball field was built, and by the end of the movie, it looked like every car in the state had lined up on the road to visit the ball field. Those days of veterinary medicine are over. No longer will the client lines appear and wait for the average practice to offer average veterinary care. The days of competitive practices and substitute sources are upon the profession.

Sources of New Clients

There are no longer many options for new clients. A new client is one of three categories: a new pet owner who has never accessed veterinary care before; an established pet owner who has just moved to town; or a pet owner who is not fully satisfied with his/her last veterinary encounter. When a potential client calls your practice, he/she wants to be assured that your practice will provide appropriate care in a timely manner, with empathy for both client and pet, while charging only an appropriate fee.

Before looking at the effectiveness of the available methods, we first must understand how clients pick practices by location. Repeated surveys report that about 60 percent of all new clients look at location first when seeking a veterinary practice; 60 percent of those selecting by location select the final choice by word of mouth referral. Again, there are only a few options available for discussion when exploring the *how:*

Word of mouth
Outside signage
Yellow pages
Professional referral
Internet linkages
Paid media
Unpaid media

The Balance of the Attraction

Some practices do not invest in their outside signage. It looks like an afterthought. A sign that is perpendicular to the street is 85 percent more effective than a sign which is attached to the front of the building. In an average practice in an average community, less than 10 percent of the new clients now come from the signage, but there are communities/locations where this "sign draw" exceeds 30 percent. A feline practice in Georgia developed a very special sign to easily denote their "feline exclusive" services and tripled their sign impact on drawing new clients. The sign must be easily read and understood in about three seconds by the passing driver. Don't overload it with information and small elements or a complicated logo. A smart practice also understands that the facility appearance and parking lot are part of their signage. An unkempt parking lot or poorly maintained exterior facade tends to make the client perceive a disorganized or unkempt practice and might cause the client to drive by and seek the next practice.

When the telephone book (yellow pages) marketing effort is assessed, community standards play a major part in the initial decision for entry level. The impact is a practice query responsibility. To judge the appropriate column space (cost), remember, a 4 to 1 ratio is needed between the money made and the money expended due to the media effort. Most practices operate on less than a 25 percent net before ROI (return on investment), which is why the 4 to 1 ratio is required. When someone says they came in because of the telephone book listing, a practice must ask why. Sometimes it is due to services, other times it may be due to a doctor's reputation, but often it is because someone has referred them to the doctor, practice, or location. This someone needs to be thanked, so the aware practice asks who.

The satisfied client who refers a friend or neighbor to a practice accounts for about 60 percent of the new clients in a quality veterinary facility. The referring clients deserve to be recognized because, as most mothers know, behavior rewarded is behavior repeated. This recognition should be at least a thank you note in the mail. If you provide an additional value-added benefit, such as movie or zoo tickets or a practice credit, supplemental reinforcement will occur. This new client will forgive more "bad day errors" than the other sign or yellow page derived new clients.

A special type of word of mouth is the professional referral. This includes pet stores, breeders, and feed stores, as well as other veterinary facilities if you have a special interest capability or special equipment. As before, behavior rewarded is behavior repeated, and some form of appreciation should be forthcoming following the referral. Some practices believe in this enough to have a special party for the best referral sources every six months, just to celebrate and say thanks. Sometimes they even share the new program introductions during this party, but that is another story.

One method sweeping the United States is use of the media to find the practice clients. Sometimes this is a newspaper ad or a radio spot, and in some other situations, it is coupons and special offers. Again, like telephone book marketing, the trend of the community is married with the practice philosophy to establish the appropriate level. Regardless, as with telephone book advertising, a 4 to 1 ratio is needed between the money made and money expended due to the media effort. The real problems with the paid media and coupon system are that the clients produce a very low net (if any), which violates the 4 to 1 ratio rule, and they show a very low rate of return to the practice (less than 25 percent). This area must be tracked for effectiveness.

The area of most fun, to me, is unpaid media exposure. There is one practice which sponsors a "meals on wheels" for pets whose owners are unable to feed them (in the hospital, shut-ins without income, etc.). This practice gets a lot of free media coverage just for the human interest of the subject. There are veterinarians who sponsor (at cost) the Scouts (or 4-H, FFA, etc.) by offering a fall rabies clinic for the community, at some central location arranged and advertised by the Scouts. This is very cheap goodwill, and it gets great, no cost, media coverage. There are many other ways, including a pet column in a local newspaper or a local pet radio hour on a Saturday or Sunday morning, to get free media coverage. All it takes is innovation and an awareness of the community needs and desires.

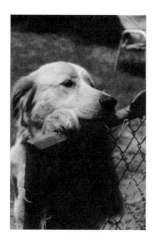

The Best Program

There is no best program. In veterinary practice, as in the stock market, another famous gambling arena, the mix-and-match always exceeds the single investment. It is a combination of the lateral actions of other practices, practice philosophy, community substitutes, and pet owner perceptions. It is also dynamic, changing frequently, often quarterly, often by the season of the year. The practice must adopt whatever programs it needs to keep the level of new clients at about 10 to 15 percent of all transactions. Most communities in America average about 20 percent pet owner movement each year, lending validity to three yardstick premises:

- When the new client access rates are higher than 15 percent, it tends to make me look for clients who fail to return.
- When the new client rate is less than 10 percent, it often indicates a low new client access rate.
- When a new client rate is less than 5 percent, it usually means the practice is dying, but it is seldom seen from inside the practice—excuses abound!

There is no great science to the method or madness associated with gathering new client information. If you want to know what attracted them to your practice, *ask them.* It is amazing what you can learn when you ask a question and then just listen. The choice for your practice is yours. Make it an overt decision.

Time Management

*An appointment is a contract, and must be kept—**on time!***

In these days of tight budgets and a demanding economy, the veterinarian's responsibility to the community must be balanced with a commitment to family, friends, and a personal quality of life. In the United States, this has led to tighter appointment schedule policies and less catering to the walk-in client. It has spawned emergency clinics that operate evenings and weekends and are supported by multiple practices. In many metroplex veterinary practices, the simple addition of "walk-ins welcomed" to the yellow page ad increases the client access rate by 25 percent; with high density schedules (shown later), this workload demand increase can be absorbed. But we will focus on only one element: the veterinary practice's office hours.

During the past decade, the average work week decreased from about 80 hours to 49 hours for most veterinarians (many new graduates complain rightly about being required to perform a 40-hour work week). We see this as a healthy trend, but it requires a change in attitude and operational habits. The majority of practicing veterinarians continually report they do not have enough leisure time. Yet we see many practitioners open earlier, stay later, and expand to weekend appointment hours. The six-day work week is *still* the norm.

Service Is an Obligation

Veterinarians are a caring lot and go out of their way to tend to the needs of their clients and patients. The same fact is true of most every member of a practice staff. That is why we entered the profession. I don't know of anyone who entered veterinary medicine primarily to become a millionaire. The expanding clinical hours in the veterinary practice community has been a response to the public demand; it is also one way to increase the income compared to a semi-fixed expense category (facility overhead). When most urban and suburban families are dual wage earners or single parents, the need for evening and weekend convenience is evident. When located in a metroplex, a morning drop-off service is a market niche based on service.

Appointment Systems

There is legislation pending in some states to address the staffing of veterinary facilities "after hours." This will be a financial challenge in the future of our profession. The use of an appointment system is still evolving. The walk-in system generally gave way to 15–30-minute appointments a decade ago, and the 20-minute appointment became commonplace by the end of the 1980s. Now the flexible 10-minute appointment log has been reintroduced to allow tailoring of the practice's appointment times. There are still a few walk-in practices, and some appointment-only practices have adopted a friendlier stand for walk-ins, using their inpatient team to handle this client need. But that is another story of better staff utilization, better held for another time.

To highlight some of the benefits of the 10-minute flexible scheduling, as discussed in the instruction sheet attached: 10 minutes for recheck or suture removal, 20 minutes for outpatient sick call, an extra 10 minutes for new clients to discuss practice philosophy, an extra 10 minutes for a second animal, an extra 10 minutes to discuss husbandry for an exotic patient, an extra 10 minutes as a senior citizen "benefit" in lieu of a discount, or even, the extra time needed for a new graduate to do anything. Using these general guidelines to develop the practice's appointment program is essential, but the real secret lies in "high density scheduling" for the doctor.

High Density Scheduling

In high density scheduling, the doctor and outpatient nurse work as a team. They have two or three consultation (exam) rooms, and *no one* is allowed to divert the nurse from supporting the doctor in these two/three rooms. With another nurse, the doctor can cover three/four consultation rooms. High density scheduling is based on overlapping the last 10 minutes of one appointment in one room with the first 10 minutes of the next appointment in the other room. The staggered schedule allows the outpatient nurse to load the other room and do the 3- to 5-minute asymmetry screen 10 minutes before the end of the pre-ceding appointment, put the record with findings on a rack outside the rear door of the exam room, then return to the room with the doctor. When the nurse enters, the doctor knows it is time to disengage and transfer the client education and close out to the nurse, *immediately!* Then the doctor moves to the other room, reviewing the wellness screen that was recorded in the medical record by the outpatient nurse and left on the rear door of the examination room.

Marketing Advantages of High Density Scheduling

As yellow page advertising and media marketing increased, quality practices centered on service to differentiate their facilities in the eyes of clients. Phrases like, "evening hours," "emergencies welcomed any time", "walk-ins welcomed," "VISA, MC, American Express, and Discover," "weekend hours," and other improved client-access factors appeared. This was very effective for the well-informed or well-bonded clients, but the less-bonded and poorly informed clients still pursued cost savings with vigor. Interestingly, the lower end (discount-type) practices have been most susceptible to failure during the recent recession. For the first time in history, the 1990s saw veterinary practices closing in response to hard times (reportedly at a 10 percent rate in Toronto, Colorado Springs, Oregon, etc.).

The annual Pfizer client research shows that Saturday hours are still the most popular, but as more practices offer early evening hours, the pressures of Satur-day are being shifted to 5:00 P.M. to 8:00 P.M. during the week (second most pop-ular time) and to Sunday hours. While this is not all bad, the tendency during these hectic appointment times is to treat the problem and not the patient. The need for return visits is overlooked, the more intensive diagnostics are waived or deferred, and some concurrent or underlying problems are never addressed. Shifting away from quality veterinary healthcare costs the practice net income, even if it increases the gross due to volume. There are options available, even with only two-doctor scheduling:

First Week	Mon	Tues	Wed	Thur	Fri	Sat	Sun
First Doctor:	7-5	11-8	off	7-5	7-7	7-2	off
Second Doctor:	10-7	7-5	7-7	11-8	off	off	off
Second Week	Mon	Tues	Wed	Thur	Fri	Sat	Sun
First Doctor:	10-7	7-5	7-7	11-8	off	off	off
Second Doctor:	7-5	11-8	off	7-5	7-7	7-2	off
			or				
	Mon	Tues	Wed	Thur	Fri	Sat	Sun
New Doctor:	off	11-8	off	11-8	8-6	7-3	off
Single Owner:	7-7	7-5	7-7	7-5	off	off	off

In the latter case, the new associate is given *four* "party" evenings a week, as well as weekday access to ski runs, beaches, hiking trails, malls, and shopping during minimal tourist/family traffic times; the single owner who has been work-ing 24/7 for years is now rewarded with three-day weekends to get to know his/her family again. The best aspect of this "new associate" schedule is that the new doctor has the *highest* productivity times, so with high density scheduling, they can derive $1500 to $2000 in personal production each day (that is $6000 to $8000 per week, or $300,000 to $400,000 per year, which at 20% productivity pay does well to pay school debts). Our consulting firm works with the VPC Brokerage to prepare practices and owners to have "smarter" hours when employing new associates, and we use the same type of leverage-the-doctor-time logic as we assist in placing practice administrators in the larger or specialty practices.

There are companion animal practices established with appointment hours only from noon to 8:00 P.M. They support a bedroom community of commuters. There are practices which have morning appointments until 10 A.M. and do not schedule appointments again until after 3 P.M.; surgery is a mid-day activity, as are mobile home calls. New companion animal veterinary facilities are being built with an odd number of exam rooms, so the doctor-nurse pairs can work two rooms, and the odd room can be used by the inpatient team to see walk-ins and emergencies in a timely manner, without disrupting the high density scheduling. This is supporting an emerging business factor, seen during this past decade: the single veterinarian practice has all but disappeared, except in start-up situations. Companion animal practices are averaging 2.6 veterinarians per facility.

Compounding these scheduling problems has been the inherent fear of client fee resistance, usually unfounded (except for quotables) in an established practice. As a rule, during the 1990s, veterinary practices found their gross slightly increasing, but their net was often decreased. The client's ability and willingness to pay for services has been put to the test, practices have raised their fees, and the average transaction charge has been rising. The ability and willingness appear to have been veterinarian based and not client demanded. The smarter practices have developed discharge planning programs that increase the client return rate rather than the average transaction fee. More "smaller ticket" visits over a period of time support the perception of lower costs; it is the client/patient return rate, not infamous average client transaction (ACT), that makes veterinary practices successful.

The greatest "demand" for extended hours is competition from other practices. The United States and Canada have increased the number of graduates during the past decade, and almost every animal owner now has multiple veterinarians to select from when they need local veterinary healthcare services. For this reason, the fear is real. If you close Saturday, the clients will find a different practice. If you take a vacation without a relief veterinarian, clients go elsewhere, and some never return. In communities without competition, Saturday hours are less important. If you are the only game in town, you set the table rules!

To get a multi-veterinarian practice into a quality of life program, we use a basic prototype of a two-week scheduling cycle for the professional staff. As shown above, the starting sequence for planning is two days on, one off, three days on, one off, four days on, then a three-day weekend. The second veterinarian starts the same schedule, but a week later. In a two doctor practice, this single staffs the practice on Friday, Saturday, and Sunday, but double staffs it on Monday, Tuesday, and Thursday (Wednesday is church night in many communities, so we recommend not fighting it); high density scheduling resolves the lower access seen with linear scheduling. The double staffing days allow for evening hours because one veterinarian can come in later (e.g., 1:00 P.M.) and work until 7:00 or 8:00 P.M. with evening appointment hours.

The bottom line is that we are a caring and dedicated profession, a group of healthcare professionals that respond to the obligation which started with Noah tending the animals on the ark. The obligation to serve must be matched to the obligation to live (or sleep in the case of farm calls), and the compromise is a personal decision. As the profession expands, the need to cooperate with our competing colleagues will outweigh the need to draw clients away. Be the first in your area to generate professional conversation concerning meeting the community's needs through rotating office hours. Meeting the needs of clients while meeting the needs of your staff and yourself will be important in the latter years of this decade.

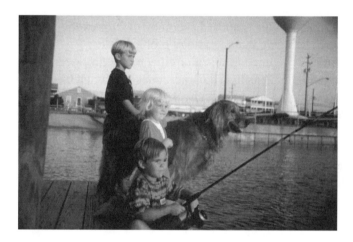

Veterinary Practice Effectiveness Begins with the Appointment Log
The Geography

- If you cannot make your computer do high density scheduling, call your vendor. For a written example, review the *Signature Series Systems & Schedules* monograph at www.v-p-c.com.
- The "surgery" column allows the client and patient to be scheduled for an early morning arrival (before 7:55 A.M.).
- The "drop-offs" column is for early arrivals, whether they are early appointments, drop-offs, or day care (insert your own times as desired).
- Most practices have core appointment hours within the 9 A.M. to 6 P.M. period, with some form of staggered lunch break.
- There are appointments over the lunch break (usually single staffed with a doctor), so use the full width if lunch time appointments are desired.
- The ". . . 5-minute" schedule endings cause far greater client compliance in arriving on time since it sounds so exact (please don't disappoint them).

- The after-7:00 P.M. appointment needs could be scheduled into the "call back" columns (times inserted as desired).
- With 2.6 doctors per clinic, the third "doctor" column can be for technician out-patient time (nutritional, parasite, dental, behavior, etc.).
- Ensure 10 minutes are blocked each two hours across both columns as "emergency space" for the client who wants to be "seen today." It is enough time to admit for day care, regardless of the reason (or it serves as coffee time or catch-up for the doctor when not scheduled).

The Schedule

[Initially discussed in *Building the Successful Veterinary Practice: Programs & Procedures* (volume 2).] After guidance, this should be the front staff's duty (not the doctors').

- A standard "sick call," with a full doctor's consultation, for an established client, is seen as 20 minutes (two spaces).
- A practice can add 10 minutes to the "standard appointment" for exotic pets, a second animal, each new client, an ophthalmology problem, etc.
- An extra 10 minutes can be scheduled as a senior citizen benefit. Social time is often more critical to senior citizens than the traditional 10 percent discount.
- A single 10-minute space can be used for recheck, suture removal, vaccine clinic, heartworm screening clinic, etc.
- Add 10 or 20 minutes to each appointment for a new graduate, only 10 extra after 90 days, and no extra "orientation" time after six months.
- Nonavailability of doctors is monitored by the receptionist team, and the log is annotated (long lunch, surgery, late arrival, early departures, etc.).

Dr.:_____　Nurse:

	Exam #1					Exam #2			
Time	Client's Name	Patient	Concern	Phone	Time	Client's Name	Patient	Concern	Phone
7:55					7:55				
8:05		New	Client		8:05				
8:15					8:15		Cat	Vac	
8:25		sick	dog		8:25				
8:35					8:35		Two	Dogs	
8:45					8:45				
8:55		Sick	Puppy		8:55				
9:05					9:05				
9:15				"E"	9:15				"E"
9:25		Sick	Dog		9:25				
9:35					9:35		Sick	Cat	
9:45		Dog	Vac		9:45				
9:55					9:55		Three	Cats	
10:05					10:05				
10:15	Elderly	Client	w/Cat		10:15				
10:25					10:25				
10:35				"E"	10:35				"E"
10:45		Cat			10:45				
10:55					10:55		Dog		
11:05		Dog			11:05				
11:15					11:15		Dog		
11:25		Cat			11:25				
11:35					11:35		Cat		
11:45		Cat			11:45				
11:55					11:55				

Table 3.1. High density scheduling example

4

Practice Programs

PROGRAMS = NET INCOME
You can only take home the net!

THIS CHAPTER is an introduction to the appendices, and it is up to the practice to pick and choose among the programs to make practice life more fun again. Yes friends, practice can be and *should be* fun; that is why we entered this very special profession. As I was surfing the net (AOL and NOAH), I watched veterinarians discuss their increase in gross, the percentage of gross that was due to vaccines or dentistry, and other such "first liar loses" type discussions. When are we going to learn? The secret of practice success lies in celebrating the human animal bond with clients, not in comparing numbers on the Internet.

The Front Door Must Swing: The Fundamentals

The secret is what makes *your* front door swing. Every practice has a different formula, but there are common components, and they are called programs (as in program-based budgeting). We realize that a preanesthetic laboratory screen is *required* in virtually every case (although the intensity and scope vary), and as stated in a recent Nevada State Board letter, 80 percent of the surgery cases should have fluids running. (When was the last time you took a fluid therapy refresher for CE?) We have stressed the grades of dental conditions and the recording of these grades in the medical records to the point where those doing it have doubled their income. We even have practices who contact Dr. Marv Samuelson (Veterinary Allergy Reference Laboratory) for assistance in developing dermatology as an income center program (e.g., even in Colorado, 15 percent of the dogs coming in the front door have atopy).

Surgical Cases

But let's go forward with fundamentals and see what you are taking for granted, especially in surgical cases. We know in our hearts that preanesthetic blood screening is essential. One state board has publicly informed every practitioner in the state that 80 percent of surgery cases should be on fluids. We read about pain management and listen to seminars, yet we believe clients can make a knowledgeable decision about pain management with no training—postsurgical pain killers are not optional—everyone knows *pain is inhumane!* Yet every day, there are practitioners putting animals at risk, and themselves into liability, by practicing "wallet medicine" instead of quality medicine.

Radiology

How about radiology? It is a fact that most practices have forgotten that a radiographic baseline of the thorax is good medicine. A boarder who is coughing does not always have kennel cough. Dogs do have other problems. For instance, a negative Difil test tells you about circulating microfilaria, not about adult heartworms in the thorax. Current literature shows that some of the coughing cats previously diagnosed as asthmatic are actually heartworm infested, even in nonendemic areas. *Only* an X ray can effectively differentiate these two conditions. Consider this: Dr. Bob Smith (radiologist, University of California, Davis) believes that dogs with a negative *or* positive heartworm test still deserve a thoracic X-ray series before starting the preventive care or treatment protocol. Moving on to the abdomen, when was the last time you did an IVP or cystogram? There are more things than just foreign bodies occurring in the abdomen. Have you ever considered the diagnostic advantage of a Baro-spheres when doing a laparotomy, since leakage is not a by-product of these pellets? During a recent short course, it was stated, "Use of the Penn Hip technique to aid in the diagnosis of hip dysplasia and the introduction of Baro-spheres for barium studies have proven diagnostic advantages." One of our clients attended and *knew* he could go back to practice and virtually double their income in this area.

Cardiac Evaluation

Look at the advances in cardiac evaluation. The handheld ECG that gives a lead-II rhythm strip can be used with every annual life-cycle consultation (yes, I know you call it an annual exam, but which sounds more accurate?). The handheld ECG is economical enough that if it were used for each "annual," at a fee of $2.00 additional, it would be totally paid for in less than six months; then it is a *net-net* program every time it is used! The use of echocardiology is on the rise; within five years most quality practices will be using it regularly. This modality is technique-driven and relatively easy to read; the difficulty lies in determining where and how to place the transducer. As Dr. Larry Tillet states so often, "Telemedicine now allows a practice to be in contact with a specialist—even across the country—within minutes."

Blood Pressure Diagnostics

Reflect on the blood pressure diagnostics of your practice. It cannot be emphasized enough. Every practice should be using a blood pressure device daily (e.g., Doppler). It has been shown that 60-plus percent of the cats in renal failure can have hypertension. It has also been shown that hypertension can be manifested in such unusual signs as anisocoria. Dr. Mike Garvey (AMC, NY) has stated that blood pressure measurement is paramount for more than hypertension—up to

30 animals die every day from hypotension for every animal that dies from hypertension.

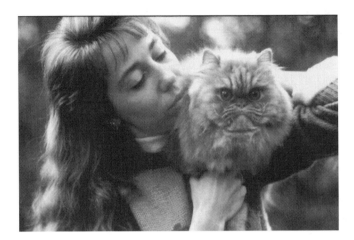

Economics

"Tom Cat, we will damage our relationship if we add these unneeded diagnostics." You are right, if they are unneeded. But in every case stated above, there was a medical need. The fact that you have taken radiology for granted means the overhead is still larger than the income from the program center. Yes, program center—not income center, not profit center. The front door swings because we believe in our healthcare programs and share that conviction with clients as *needs* for their animal(s). If you don't medically believe it is needed, *never* do it!

And for those of you who take one film to "save the client money," remember what every text and radiologist has stated, "If it looks like a duck, sounds like a duck, and walks like a duck, it must be considered a duck . . . and ducks state very clearly, *quack, quack, quack!*" If radiology is needed, two views are needed. To provide half the care is a violation of professional ethics and the Practice Act. Think of lameness cases where you have said, "If this does not get better, we may need to take radiographs." The client brought a suffering animal to you because he/she wanted peace of mind, but you only offered "tincture of time." And you wonder why they never come back! Lameness generally requires radiology to determine the appropriate treatment as well as the prognosis.

The ability to believe in good medicine is the cornerstone of a successful practice. The ability to convey this need to clients is the cornerstone of a profitable practice. The overhead of a veterinary practice is pretty fixed (in well-managed practices, less than 50 percent of the gross income is spent on monthly expenses, not counting rent, doctor monies, and ROI benefits). So, it is the delivery of services and products within existing staff and facility capabilities that can make the net income difference.

Choices for the Future

We really don't care what you have already done; that is past. What we care about is what you are willing to do. Every year, new continuing education courses mean you have the opportunity to enhance practice programs. The continuing education experience that does not add one new program per day of CE attended is a wasted expense. The Shirt Sleeve Seminars, conducted by Veterinary Practice Consultants *(www.v-p-c.com),* are designed to be economical weekend programs for staff and doctors; the energy levels seen when staff get to plan the programs to promote the human-animal bond is exciting to experience (and very profitable when they are supported). The new programs need to be designed to provide better care, and there is a value associated with that client benefit. That value, as assessed to clients, should be reflected in your program-based budget for the year. The cash flow reports from that computer in your office *only* reflect the "belief level" of the providers in the new program(s) being offered. The choice is yours; we are here to help, but the belief starts in your gut and ascends to your heart. When your heart believes in the program, clients will accept the care as needed and essential. It is your choice—lower the net each year, or provide better healthcare delivery programs.

Communicating to Win

> *The man who will use his skill and constructive imagination to see how much he can give for a dollar, instead of how little he can give for a dollar, is bound to succeed.*
>
> —Henry Ford

PetsMart, Wal-Mart, and even the grocery store down the street have decided to offer alternatives to the clients of your practice. They are competing for the pet healthcare dollar. Some even hire corporations that provide low-cost veterinarians. What the competition does not have is a technician-veterinarian healthcare delivery team to *listen to the clients;* listening is a way to become "special" in the client's mind. The veterinarian may produce the gross income, but the technician can produce the net income required for survival and prosperity. In a progressive veterinary practice, together you offer a caring and trusted alternative to concerned pet owners—*if they choose to talk to you.*

Getting and Giving Information

> *The worse the news, the more effort should go into communicating it.*
>
> —A.S. Grove

Communication is simply the getting and giving of information. When a consumer enters an average retail store, it is "buyer beware." When they enter a "discount store," it is different. They expect less quality and better prices and look forward to finding a bargain from some standard they have preestablished in their mind. The communication that occurs is usually price centered. When a healthcare consumer enters a healthcare facility, that person is stressed, but there is still an expectation of quality service at a fair price. There is also an unspoken social contract that exists in healthcare settings:

• First, the veterinary healthcare facility team will do no harm.
• Secondly, the providers will only do what is needed.
• Thirdly, there will be a fair fee assessed for the services rendered.
• Fourth, all parties want to restore wellness in the patient.

In the examination room, most veterinarians speak in professional terms, which is appropriate if explained; however, explanations seldom occur. Most clients don't know about the most common terms (e.g., FVRCP, DHLAPP, FeLV, FIV, etc.,) and understand less about the -itis, -osis, -ectomy, and even "benign" findings. (A recent survey by the American College of Healthcare Executives showed 46 percent of the population did not understand the term "benign" when used with the word "cancer.")

Clients deserve to be told what is needed and why. They deserve the opportunity to ask questions. They deserve the respect of the healthcare provider. When these steps have been taken, the client needs to be asked for his/her position. The phrase may be, "What seems fair for your pet today?" . . . or . . . "Do you want us to start today, or would you like to make an appointment for a return visit?" or some other positive request for a positive reply. I do not advocate levels of care, just alternative "yes" replies. When a "maybe," a "stall" or a question is the reply, then we react in accordance with the situation. Regardless of the reply, client bonding requires that we take the 30 to 60 seconds needed to validate the client's decision. This short effort gets the client back through the door. This is positive communication.

Sharing the Burden

Speech is a mirror of the soul; as a man speaks, so he is.
—Publilius Syrus

The first response to the communication emphasis discussed in the paragraph above is, "There isn't enough time in the day!" Does that mean you don't want clients to come back, or does it mean you don't want clients to be supportive of the treatment plan offered? There are alternatives to the doctor doing all the examination room "communication." In most veterinary practices in America, there exists at least one underutilized staff member waiting to be developed. Doctors try to do too much themselves and, in turn, don't do enough for each client and pet. Ask yourself these questions:

• Who does the nutritional counseling?
 - Are there serial weights, with body scores, in every medical record?
 - Who does the monthly client recall, patient appearance recheck, and weigh-ins?
 - Who monitors the client's reorder point for prescription diets?
 - Who discusses the home supplementation concerns when the client stops the prescription diet feeding?
• Who does the parasite prevention and control counseling?
 - Does the practice understand the difference between foggers and a premises eradication guarantee (such as FLEABUSTERS)?

- Who actually defines where in the house (floor plan assessments) foggers need to go for most effect versus a total premises plan?
- Who does the follow-up to ensure there was effective elimination?
- Who ensures the external parasite and internal parasite relationships (e.g., tapeworms, anemia, etc.) are understood by the client?

• Who does the dental hygiene counseling?
- Are there serial dental grades (1+ to 4+) in every medical record?
- Are clients allowed to go home and are they asked to rub the pet's teeth nightly with tuna water (cats) or garlic water (dogs) before coming back to discuss dental options? Who does this return visit counseling?
- Who takes the time to discuss the diet and bad breath effects of poor teeth?
- Who cares enough to tell clients that "red gums mean pain" and explain the healthcare options?

• Who does the behavior management counseling?
- Does it *automatically* start with the puppy/kitten series?
- Is house training assistance given during the first puppy/kitten visit as a value-added service?
- Who spends time listening to the client's needs (85 percent report that they do have a pet behavior problem)?
- Who schedules short familiarization times in the clinic on a weekly basis to help change the unwanted behavior?
- Who does the callbacks to ensure the behavior management ideas are working in the home with all the family members?

• Who does the client callbacks?
- New clients are called and told, *"Welcome to our practice!"*
- Postmedication dispensing call (half-way through treatment) to ensure client does not have questions (and hasn't stopped the treatment program or forgotten the recheck appointment).
- Postsurgical call, at recovery and again four days after discharge, to ensure the client has no worries.
- To promote the human-animal bond, *and* to "walk the talk," any deferred or symptomatic care *must* receive increased surveillance until the condition is resolved. Nursing staff must ensure the client does not have questions and knows to return when things are not going as planned; nurses can even do the interim recheck appointment.

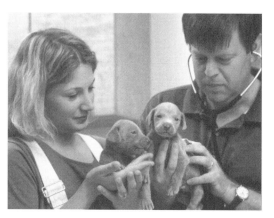

The above examples are just a few situations where the receptionist-technician team members can extend the effectiveness of the veterinarian. Veterinary extenders may also be reminder postcards, established staff protocols, laboratory result telephone calls to the client, or a host of other client service oriented activities. A client should perceive a higher level of service and caring when he/she contacts a veterinary hospital (the pet health expert in the community), and in most practices, 80 percent of these contacts have traditionally been with the paraprofessional staff. It is the caring and knowledge of the technician and receptionist that allow the client to form that "first impression" and "practice image."

Client Communications

Informing the Client

> *Man is a dog's ideal of what God should be.*
> —Holbrook Jackson

The veterinarian's charge goes back to Noah—the Lord said to tend to the animals of the land. It is the responsibility of the veterinary healthcare team to speak for the needs of the animals we care for—to be their advocate! Concurrently, we must give the client the right to make an informed decision, which means we should take the time to explain the animal's needs and, on many occasions, the alternatives available to meet those needs. The higher the client's knowledge of the healthcare needs (veterinary IQ), the more often the animal will receive the needed care. The patient advocate ensures the client is aware of the what is needed to restore or maintain wellness and allows the client to make an informed decision.

The patient advocate desires the best care possible, but the budget of the household often can afford only part of what is needed during any given pay period (proof of this is in your own paycheck each pay period). It is the paraprofessional healthcare provider who can keep contact with the client and negotiate a return next month for some of the other care needed. The enthusiasm and caring of the technician or receptionist can help make this return decision a practice reality. When a staff member becomes a healthcare team member, client communications improve. Many clients feel more comfortable discussing concerns with the technician because (1) they don't want to take the doctors time, (2) they don't understand the terms he/she uses, or simply, (3) they feel it is easier to talk to the technician or the receptionist. The client's concern must be answered first if the practice wants to keep the client returning, and the client's concern (patient's problem) is first told to a staff member, not the doctor. This is why the staff member has such a great influence on the number of clients entering a practice. The urgency or need is established with the first contact.

The nurse technician team needs to work with the client relations reception team to ensure that the narratives and understanding exist about every practice program and service. When a client calls about a flea or tick problem, is there an urgency? Can't fleas and ticks be handled with a bath and some dusting powder from a pet store? What level of in-service education has been conducted for the staff members at your hospital? Do they know the other diseases for which the animal needs to be screened in a tick or flea case (e.g., Lyme disease, tapeworms, etc.) and how to best communicate this need to clients? Some veterinary practices have initiated a "technician hot line" just to ensure the client can reach someone who has the time to care. What are the client education skills your practice has developed within the staff members who talk to clients on the phone, at the front desk, or in the exam room? How are they reinforced? Who is the patient advocate?

Listening to the Client

It takes two to speak the truth—one to speak and one to hear.
—Thoreau

Clients are not well informed consumers of veterinary healthcare services. They do not understand the levels of quality and training that are so variable between the suppliers available. As a profession, we haven't helped this situation that much. We still deal in "quotables" on a daily basis. Communicating to win is not selling a service or product. It is letting people buy. Look at the world around you. People are not sold newspapers, they are buying information (or comics, or sports). You don't want to be sold circus tickets; you want to buy the thrills and entertainment. When someone parks a new car in his/her driveway, the first statement is, "Look at the neat car I just *bought*," but when something goes wrong, the phrase becomes, "Look at the lemon they *sold* me!"

If we assume listening to the clients is a given (which it seldom is), then we meet their needs and wants *first*. In veterinary healthcare, during the physical examination we often discover additional patient needs that must be prioritized into the care plan. Communicating to win has four basic steps that any practice can learn to follow:

1. Make the client aware of a *preexisting* condition that needs attention.
2. Educate the client about the changes in the veterinary profession that now allow us to address the condition.
3. With caring and enthusiasm, offer your practice's program to address the client's concern (patient's problem).
4. After the client replies, validate the response, regardless of what it is, and set the expectation for the next encounter.

Be ready for the client to ask the basic buying questions: What is it? Why do I need it? How much is it? Is it really needed now? What is the value to me? As you can see, the client bases most decisions on the *emotion* of the moment, while the average veterinary practice addresses the *logic* of the need. Logic will seldom answer the emotional need, but staff members who care can! The pet owner wants to know how much you care, not how much you know. Clients expect professional excellence when they contact a veterinarian's office, so don't disappoint them by recommending a "tincture of time" brush-off. They also want the caring, so never disappoint them in this area!

The opening contact with a client is a time to gather information and should be nonthreatening (avoid questions that require only a "yes" or "no" answer). A "phone shopper" should be mailed a hospital brochure, newsletter, or flyer the same day of the call, so an address is also an important piece of information.

You need to stress that you treat the whole animal and care for the whole family, not just one part of the animal. When healthcare recommendations are made, they need to be stated as "needs." Be clear about the needs of the animal and the needs of the practice. For instance, a preanesthesia laboratory profile is a professional need so we can ensure there isn't something going on that we cannot see that may cause anesthetic complications. There is a need to explain the entire wellness approach of the practice. Health is an entire project, for animals as well as for their owners.

After the low-key conversational greeting, the information gathering, and the evaluation of total wellness, the client must make the decision to buy. If the smart technician or receptionist offers two "yes" alternatives, the ability to "buy" is assisted. The best way for someone to *close a sale* varies with the service, the product, and the individuals involved within the discussion. There is no one best way. Regardless of the closure method, one additional step is needed. A caring practice will ensure it *comforts the buying decision.* Whether the client has opted for full service, partial care, deferred service, or simply waived the care, the client must feel comfortable with the decision if you want a return to the practice another time. Return visits make a greater net for the practice than the search for new clients, so to establish the expectation for their next visit is part of the "comforting" action. If the dental decision was ". . . not today . . .," assign a technician to the client/patient and set expectations for the telephone follow-up to ensure the "red gums (red = pain)" are resolved. You accept the clients and their decisions, and you want to see them again!

These ideas do not guarantee success, they only allow you to add to the practice's success. How you approach client service and patient care will make the difference. How the practice empowers the staff to extend the veterinary caring will make a difference, but the caring delivered by you will be the real difference.

Educating the Client

Education makes people easy to lead but difficult to drive.

Most veterinarians find themselves giving a standard set of instructions to their clients concerning common animal problems. It is usually repetitious, monotonous, and time consuming for both the practitioner and the client (who may even perceive the boredom in the doctor's presentation). It is usually all too soon forgotten. There are better ways to inform the client about conditions and concerns, more effective methods to ensure retention of important information, and most important, proven techniques to decrease the monotony and time involved in conducting "client education."

Effective educational tools can ease the burden on the practitioner in the exam room, strengthen client appreciation and referrals, and expand the market for veterinary services— if—the message is delivered by an informed and caring staff member.

For many veterinarians, printed and audiovisual client education materials appear to be the answer. Indeed, most practitioners already rely on some form of instructional material in addition to verbal advice, but in an inconsistent manner.

The staff member must be added to the equation to make any "system" effective. With careful thought, preparation, and some investment, the right type of client education material can be an effective practice builder resulting in client appreciation and referrals. Every veterinarian and staff member needs to weigh the benefits of expanding the practice's client education resources and delivery methods against the cost of producing and/or acquiring the material to be used. The benefit analysis should include consideration of the following:

- *Saving Time.* In the United States, less than 10 percent of the practices never distribute tailored educational material of any kind. Most practitioners agree that handing out materials that deal with common animal problems saves time and eases the monotony of repeating instructions to clients. A caution is in order though, since an overreliance on printed or audiovisual materials may cause the client-doctor bond to be broken. Clients deserve verbal communication time; less is often resented. It is best when a staff member presents the handout with a narrative that points out the key elements to ensure successful understanding.

- *Customizing.* More practices that put together their own materials often blend a few manufacturer resources with their own flyers. To add a bonding factor to the literature, these must be explained one-by-one by a caring nursing staff member. For instance, a handout titled "Traveling with Your Pet" allows a practice to identify local parasite and health problems and still warn the client of the dangers that lie outside the community environment. This customized approach is also very important following a surgery or inpatient stay since each practice has different expectations for the clients. The customizing and outreach by informed team members allows the practice to differentiate itself in the eyes of its clients, which may detract or add to the quality perception depending on the effort expended in the client education piece.

- *Client Response.* There has been a generally positive response whenever a practice has augmented its client education material, sometimes to the extent of receiving thank you notes and additional referrals. In high volume–lower price type practices, the client acceptance rate drops. Almost 40 percent of the price shoppers seem disinterested in being educated. Almost every practice that employs staff-supported client education techniques reports the procedures pay for themselves as a practice building device.

- *Access Rate.* The informed client has a greater access rate (more visits per year). It is more visits at "community standard" average client transaction (ACT) rates that bonds clients (rapidly escalating ACTs can break the client-practice bond for mid-range clients). Informed clients seem to better understand the need for preventive healthcare, as well as be more alert to signs of disease and discomfort in their pets. These clients are more likely to ask about dental hygiene, elective surgery, and parasite control.

The selection of client education material varies from practice to practice, and the better practices use a mixture of techniques to ensure there are methods compatible with the specific needs of most clients. The recurring cost may be minimal for those practices that use exclusively vendor supplied resources, or can range into the hundreds of dollars per year for those practices that customize most of their client education material. Clearly, the importance (and affordability) of client education to veterinarians differs substantially between practitioners. The basic components of a client education program are a combination of custom material (e.g., practice brochure), vendor references (e.g., vaccination literature), and audiovisual resources. There are benefits to each of the options.

- *Audiovisual.* Most practices in the United States have now changed to the videotape, audiovisual format of presentation. Some still use self-produced slide presentations. The early veterinary videotape programs were ineffective because they were too long and presented too much technical information. Clients do not need to become professionally educated, they just require an increased awareness of needs. While the initial cost for audiovisual equipment is expensive, especially with a viewing system in each exam room, the ability to utilize the systems for staff training pays for the system in saved leadership time. The selection of short (less than 10 minutes) client education videos has increased, as have the staff training video resources.

- *Practice Brochure.* This one piece of "emotional" promotional material needs to be an educational effort as well. Most clients are unaware of the scope of services, the technical expertise, or the diversity of training available in a veterinary practice. *Beware*—a brochure is not a client rule book; it needs to be a client enticement. This applies to food animal and equine as well as companion animal practices. Practices differ by more than appointment hours and location, but most clients are never told anything further. A well-illustrated practice brochure goes a long way to tell and show clients what happens "behind the scenes" in their veterinary hospital. Credit systems available, staff's special interests, and descriptions of what the practice really provides add to the usefulness of this practice building tool, but the presentation must be addressed to the feelings and emotions of the client, not just the logic of the practice.

- *Newsletters.* The regular newsletter gained popularity during the 1980's and lost favor as we entered the 1990's. This is too bad. It is a bonding activity. It provides each client with the written word to be read at leisure. The client's comprehension when "listening" to the veterinarian is generally lower than when he/she is reading similar written material. The written word has power—it can be shared with a spouse at a later date. The newsletter in a food animal practice is a very good way to increase producer awareness of changes in the industry and wellness standards that may increase yields. A "new client" newsletter could be developed and maintained at the reception desk to introduce both new clients and phone shoppers to the practice team, the practice facilities, and the practice philosophy of excellence and care.

- *Handouts.* Explanatory handouts have become critical to practice communications. Besides promotional literature from vendors, there are books of explanatory handouts available, as well as computer-driven narratives to insert into final invoices. One practice developed an "Owner's Manual" for households with new puppies and kittens that follows the format of new car booklets. Instead of "thousands of miles" between check-ups and maintenance, they used "pet ages" and got a great client response.

• *Veterinary Staff.* The delivery of *all of the above* is best done by a veterinary nurse or technician in the quiet of an examination room. This person has the client's ear, does not talk "doctor's talk" too often, and has both the compassion and the time to spend with the client. If the doctor does not routinely use an outpatient technician nurse, then the doctor is either (1) doing technician work or (2) shortchanging the client on information. Neither is profitable!

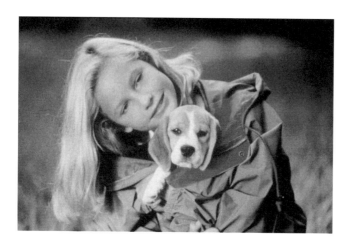

When Their Worry Appears to Be the Cost

♪ ♪ ♪ *How Much Is That Doggy in the Window . . . ?* ♪ ♪ ♪

The tail will keep wagging if we can give clients an economical way to spend their small amount of discretionary income on their pets. When clients call, they do not want to hear a laborious explanation from an untrained receptionist of why the practice's prices are so high; good pet owners want the best value for the best price. So please, answer their question directly, using ideas from the following:

Dialogues

Dialogue 1
Q: How much is a dentistry?
A: Do you have pet medical health insurance?
Q: No, why?
A: Because if you did, our adolescent dental would be less than $50 after reimbursement!

Dialogue 2
Q: How much are the annual vaccinations?
A: Do you have pet medical health insurance?
Q: No, why?
A: Because if you did, our annual booster series, with a doctor's consultation, would be less than $20 after reimbursement!

Dialogue 3

Q: I saw the Purnia Silver Pet ad about annual blood testing; what is the cost?

A: Do you have pet medical health insurance?

Q: No, why?

A: Because if you did, our full blood chemistry would be less than $20 after reimbursement!

Supplemental and Optional Statements

Since you are worried about cost, let me send you a pet insurance brochure, and if it looks right for you, please call the company. It is not practice exclusive, so if you need to use an emergency practice, or we need to refer your pet to a specialist, the insurance is still in effect.

Since you want the best price, the wellness care portion of this policy provides over two dollars of reimbursement for every dollar of premiums . . . Two dollars back for every dollar spent is the best deal on the street today! They also have monthly payment plans.

Pet insurance premiums are age dependent, so for $10 to $15 a month, you can receive coverage for sickness, injury, and wellness care, and with over $215 dollars of wellness care reimbursement available a year, even if your pet does not get sick or injured, you can receive more reimbursement that what you paid in premiums.

Bring Them in So You Can Take It to the Bank

All veterinarians work in one way or another to educate their clients. They try to educate them about preventive needs, wellness needs, and curative needs. They discuss common problems and what veterinary medicine can do for the clients' pets. Some practitioners rely solely on the spoken word, but that information deteriorates before the sun sets. That is why most successful practices have progressed to some form of literature.

> *All clients deserve the courtesy of having something educational in hand when they leave the practice, to read after they get home, when they can relax from the stress of the visit.*

Literature can be acquired from pharmaceutical and feed companies, publishers, veterinary associations, and other vendors that support our industry. They spend hundreds and thousands of dollars on sophisticated written, illustrated, and audiovisual promotions every year. Those who want to be different or desire to customize their approach to their own community can develop personalized pieces to supplement the professionally produced pieces from national organizations. There is general agreement that client education materials, at the very least, save time and money while ensuring a comprehensive delivery of information. Some assert that the additional effort expended on personalized practice brochures, newsletters, and handouts is repaid many times over by the growth of the practice and the public recognition of veterinary medicine as a healthcare profession. Regardless, the trend is to more information, not less. The client's desire is for more information, not less. The caring practice will deliver more information, not less, in a client friendly manner that does not overwhelm the animal owner.

The practice building tools presented here and in the appendices are aimed at educating the client through caring veterinary healthcare providers. But remember, strong practice leadership must focus on staff training *before* client marketing. The focus must be on the *caring* rather than on the *bottom line*.

For additional information on many of the ideas presented, see the list of related works at the front of this book.

As an example of how far the veterinary practice still has to go in patient advocacy, I'll tell you what happened when I had to take control of the healthcare of our Maine Coon cat, Merlin (see dedication).

- When Merlin reached middle age, I had to require the veterinarian who tended to Merlin when I was on the road to do a full blood chemistry; her reply to my wife was, "Yes, I should have recommended it, but most of my clients do not accept it, so I have quit mentioning it." Her belief level was lower than I ever expected.

- With a bit of extra knowledge on trends, we adjusted his diet and treated his joints; his quality of life was pretty good. When I came home, he greeted me with his "silent meows" and waited until I sat down before he head-butted me and had his ears "scritched"; he would sit next to me for hours, never invading my space, just sharing the closeness. At bedtime, when I retired to the bedroom, he would follow, jump up on the bed, walk across my body, and head-butt me until I scritched his ears as he lay at a comfortable arm's length; when I started to doze, he went back to his nightly household rounds, those things important to cats of his age and dominance.

- In the spring of last year, while I was traveling, Merlin's urine turned red, and I directed that he be taken to the same veterinarian for an immediate urinalysis and evaluation. The results were negative, the doctor told my wife, and I was called on the road; like a normal client, I know red urine is bad, so I asked about the blood chemistry and radiology. My wife asked the veterinarian and the response was, "Yes, I should have recommended it, but most of my clients do not accept it, so I have quit mentioning it." The results were negative, the doctor told my wife, and I was called on the road.

- We all know that red urine is not good, so I asked about the contrast study or ultrasound recommendations. My wife asked the veterinarian and the response was, "Yes, I should have recommended it, but most of my clients do not accept it, so I have quit mentioning it." An ultrasound with a specialist was scheduled; tumors were in the bladder and had spread throughout the colon, and Merlin's liver was very cystic; we started pain management.

- Now the veterinarian thought she was ready, so she offered chemotherapy and exploratory surgery; I explained that a 17-year-old Maine Coon cat with this extensive a metastasis was not a great candidate for heroic treatments, and we would closely manage his pain and quality of life.

- In July of last year, I came home from the AVMA annual meeting, and as I walked in the door, Merlin did his "silent meow," took a few steps towards me, and lay down; he was in pain. I asked how long he had been in pain, and my family said he had not eaten in 36 hours and had not moved much. Each member of my family is trained in some aspect of healthcare, yet they had missed his "pain" movement.

• I lay down on the floor next to Merlin, scritched his ears, and made the decision that we were at the end of pain management and he was now suffering. He was too important to me for anything less, so the decision was made to allow him to cross the rainbow bridge.

• If I had been an average client, I would have denied Merlin's pain as my family had, and maybe I would have blamed the veterinarian, or even bargained with the Lord for some extra time with this long-time friend and comrade. But I was not an average client, I am a veterinarian. I have been given responsibility for the lives of others, a covenant to tend to the animals of the land, and granted the privilege of offering a humane death in cases of undue suffering.

• Every member of my family now knows how to identify pain in animals, and every client we consult with has been asked to accept pain scoring as a standard of practice. I have always been strong on patient advocacy, and my belief in this profession is strong; I never want a client to encounter what my wife did when she took Merlin in for veterinary assistance. This book, and the support of the friends who have contributed portions to this text, is one step towards that goal.

Good clients do not follow discounts and do not want short-cuts in healthcare for their animals; they are stewards of the life of a trusted friend and will follow a caring provider. Clients deserve caring veterinary staffs, and patients deserve to have an advocate who speaks for their well-being. Caring staff members do not follow a dictator, they follow the doctor with vision and a caring heart. The appendices of this text provide concepts and ideas; they are not to be followed by rote; they require a caring leader to caress the ideas and make them their own. The focus must always be on clients; they are the stewards who need to be informed and nurtured. The informed client will want to purchase needed care and will resist being drawn away from a practice that has conveyed its caring and concern with an integrated client education program. Clients may change veterinarians when they don't know the difference, but they don't leave a veterinary practice that cares! As you embrace the bond and as your practice becomes known for the "caring heart" approach to veterinary healthcare delivery, never lose the dream, never lose the caring that caused you to select this profession; I can hope no more for any colleague or staff.

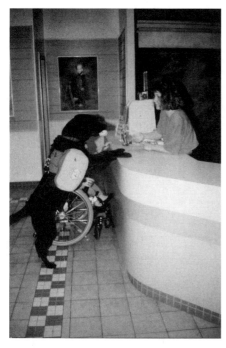

Courtesy of Lisa Ferrerio
and Delta Society.

Appendix A

Saying Thanks

$\mathbf{M}$OST OF us were taught when we were young that to say "thank you" was important. McDonald's has built a worldwide empire by saying "thanks" in many languages. Saying "thank you" is supposed to be one of the most powerful tools we have to recognize and motivate our practice staff members. In human-animal bond activities, it sets the stage and reinforces the mood. We need to find new ways to say thank you to our clients.

The First Impression

A pleasant voice on the phone and a smile when a new client arrives go a long way toward starting the client-practice bond. In many practices, new clients are then given a "client registration form"—this is slightly ahead of the "new client form." We have done many surveys, and all new clients know who they are, they just don't know who you are. The form we recommend is provided on the form diskette in the Signature Series Monograph on Systems and Schedules (at *www.v-p-c.com*), but the top looks like the following example:

WELCOME TO OUR PRACTICE ! ! !

Thank you for giving us the opportunity to care for your pet. Please help us meet your needs better by taking a moment to share some important information we will need as we support your pet's needs today and in the future. **PLEASE PRINT IN ALL SPACES**.

CLIENT'S NAME_____

SPOUSE/OTHER_____

Value-Added Thank You's

We need to say "thank you" to the new client for selecting our practice; the initial form is followed by a phone call, to the effect:

Hi, Mrs. Brown. This is Kacie at Acme Veterinary Hospital. The doctor and I wanted to say thank you for selecting us to care for Spike. We want to ensure you have not had any more questions since your visit and confirm that we are looking forward to seeing Spike again in two weeks. Do you have any questions at this time?

At some practices we even remember to say thank you to the person who sent us the new client (instead of minimal and arbitrary in-house discounts, we recommend a thank you card, an extra newsletter, or a brochure for the next referral; and after the first referral we recommend movie or zoo tickets as a "thank you" gesture—these are all tax deductible, and discounts are not). Most practices seldom use the "thank you" effort as a method to reinforce the human-animal bond or show the caring of the practice. This effort should also highlight your community commitment, specialization, or board certification. At the end of this appendix is a hospital stationary sample that shows one alternative that could be used in this effort.

The secret is to make the "thank you" a special occurrence in the life of the client. How to add something of value to the letter that makes the sender special is the task at hand. Using a client brochure—if the brochure has been made client friendly and is not the traditional "rule book" of client compliance—is only one example. A brochure is enclosed with a request to share it with another friend. On a second thank you to the same client, I often recommend using a pair of discount movie tickets since it meets the multiple-marketing impact: a gee whiz when they open the envelop, a gee whiz when they go to the show (or send the kids), and a gee whiz when someone mentions the movie and the client says, "My veterinarian sent me tickets so we went for free!"

Some "lower income client" practices prefer to offer a discount on the next visit, but this is not tax deductible, nor are discount seekers often great clients.

Sending a discount coupon to be used at the practice is often counterproductive with upper middle class clients, since it makes the gesture appear to be a sales gimmick rather than a sincere "thank you" for accessing the quality and *needed* healthcare.

The value-added target is to elevate the impression of the practice and staff in the mind of the client. The method chosen must fit the practice philosophy and the values of the practice team. Do it with the end result rather than the process of the thank you as the driving force.

Expand on That Thought

How many times do people get thanked for community or personal accomplishments? Answer: not enough!

People accomplish many things that go largely unnoticed. If you want the practice and yourself to stand out in clients' memories, send notes to acknowledge their accomplishments. Have the receptionist team screen the local newspapers for clients they remember who have made the news and let them pen the note for your signature. Be very specific and concise about the accomplishment. Do not market the practice in this note. The fact that you took the time will make the difference in the receiver's thought process.

Try to differentiate your practice by being a community advocate, saying thanks whenever someone does that "good turn" for the community or a member of the community. Again, have your staff watch the local newspaper for reasons to send congratulatory thank you notes for commendable community efforts. Let your staff pen the note, for your signature, that acknowledges their "giving" to others.

Unlike the personal accomplishment note that is usually restricted to clients, the community effort thank you notes can go to anyone in town. They can even go to anyone in the state. If you get the staff to think about recognizing others, do not hamper their zeal. Their excitement will be conveyed to the clients. Again, do not market the practice in these notes. Rather, just be a concerned citizen.

The Final Thank You

As clients depart your practice, they are usually quickly forgotten, especially if they change practices. This is one of the worst mistakes a practice can make. That client has changed practices for a reason. You may or may not know the real reason. A client transferred by his/her company might just be crossing paths with a pet owner who is coming to town to fill the vacated position. You want the referral! A courteous departure, with a "thank you for letting us care for your pet" note sent to the client's new home, will differentiate your practice. This is especially important if the client followed the "reduced price ads" to a high volume, low touch practice.

As before, the receptionist staff should compose the note as a matter of course. The signature of the veterinarian can be expanded to include the entire staff.

Regardless, let the client know that you care and that you are available for questions from the next veterinarian.

Your concern and attention to this matter is appreciated. Thank you!

Sample Letter(s)

HOSPITAL STATIONERY
* * S A M P L E * *

Dear Mrs. Jones:

This note is just to say thank you for referring someone to this practice.

—or—

This letter is to say thank you for sharing your confidence in our practice with a friend.

—or—

Thank you for referring Mrs. _____ and Fluffy to _____ Animal Hospital. We did our very best to provide responsive quality care and not disappoint them or embarrass your confidence in our practice.

—then—

Your referral came in this week, so we thought you might like to know a little more about the quality of care we believe in and the services we offer to our community. We have enclosed

—then—

a copy of our hospital brochure (OR an issue of our new client newsletter) to share with another friend or neighbor who may wish to try a new veterinary healthcare facility.

—or—

something about the national organization we voluntarily subscribe to, the American Animal Hospital Association (AAHA). We belong to the AAHA so that we can have their practice consultants perform independent, recurring, on-site evaluations of the quality of our veterinary healthcare and the quality of our facility. We want to provide the very best quality, and this is one way. We have enclosed a brochure to tell you more about the standards that we must continue to meet to remain a member of the AAHA (less than 20 percent of the veterinary hospitals in the United States are willing to undergo this level of professional evaluation).

—then a caring closure—

We hope this information will remind you of how much we care about you and your pet. Again, we thank you for your referral, and hope that your confidence in this practice's quality care will increase with every visit.

Sincerely,

Ima Friend, DVM

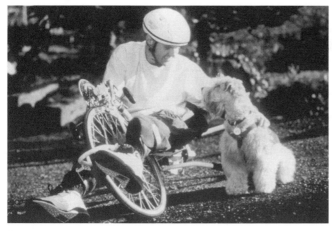

Courtesy of Frank Siteman
and Delta Society.

Appendix B

Operation Pet ID

THE FIRST week in May is National Pet Week. One year's theme was "Happiness is a Healthy Pet," and each year the AVMA Auxiliary selects a great theme promoting some aspect of the human-animal bond. Happiness is also peace of mind when it comes to a pet's security and the chances of the pet being returned if lost. We have all heard of "Operation Identification," where local police organizations and schools team together to have children photographed and fingerprinted to help locate them if they become lost or missing. Have you ever heard of "Operation Pet ID?"

As a component of your hospital's integrated business and marketing plans, the public awareness benefit of an "Operation Pet ID" could be phenomenal. With the increased media attention to animal humane issues, the AVMA Auxiliary's efforts in May, and the acceptance of the human–companion animal bond as a way of life, clients have become sensitized to the need for their pets' security and have become more concerned about the safety and protection of their pet.

Public Relations Serving Practice Promotion

Your hospital can perform a valuable public outreach program while simultaneously strengthening your client's bond to the hospital. Consider the following components for your hospital's "Operation Pet ID" program:

• Designate each Tuesday evening during the month of May as an "Operation Pet ID" night in conjunction with the annual National Pet Week campaign emphasizing pet wellness.

- Publish the dates and times in your hospital's newsletter and send press releases to the local newspapers and radio stations.
- Set up displays that inform pet owners about tattooing pets for identification, its availability, and its relative permanence, compared to ID tags. If ID implants are utilized in your area of the country, inform owners of their availability also.
- Take a photograph of the pet (with the owner, if possible) using an instant camera and affix it to your hospital's "Pet Identification Sheet."
- Record for the owner the vital information which is necessary for an accurate identification of the animal. This would include information such as breed, weight, haircoat, color tag numbers, and location of tattoo numbers.
- If the owner is a current client, make a photocopy of the sheet for the medical record. If the owner is not a client, recommend that a photocopy be provided (by the owner) to his/her veterinarian for future reference.
- Encourage the owner to review the information at least annually and update the information and the pet's picture at that time.
- Include on the reverse of the "Pet Identification Sheet" (see below) some tips for pet safety and what to do if a pet is lost. Some examples can be obtained from the AVMA's *Marketing and Practice Strategies for the Companion Animal Practice* program text.
- Remember to put your hospital's name, address, and phone number on the identification sheet.
- Provide the owners with window decals (see below) to notify firemen and emergency personnel of how many animals are inside and what to do with them. Distribute wallet sized emergency cards (see below) designed to alert authorities of the need to care for pets at home in the event of a personal accident or illness away from home. Reassure the owner that the hospital team will be there to care for the pets when necessary.

Empower Your Staff

Assign a staff member to be the program director or designate a team to oversee the program's organization. Make sure staff members know what the outcome is to be so that they can direct the proper output. Be enthusiastic. More than likely this is a first in the community, and your hospital is now a community leader. Empower the team to research specifics for your area and develop an implementation plan to maximize your hospital's public relations image.

Jointly establish a timeline for accomplishments. The program director should provide updates on a regular basis, and the entire staff should celebrate individual accomplishments as they occur.

Be ready to address the ancillary components of the program. When a client elects to have a pet tattooed and the procedure and risks associated with the anesthesia of an overweight dog are explained, the hospital's representative should be ready to discuss the alternatives for restoring the pet to the proper weight (or at least refer the client to the in-house nutritional consultant). When the owner says "I have to get this done because Phydeaux runs away a lot," be prepared to discuss the availability of behavior management aids and counseling.

When you utilize the caring personalities of your staff, this is a "win/win" program: win for the client and pet, and win for your hospital's reputation.

Pet's
Name:_____

Breed:_____

Color:_____

Haircoat:
Long Medium Short

Weight:_____

Distinctive Markings:
_____

_____

_____

photo identification here

ID Tags? YES   NO

Tag #_____

Tattoo #_____

Location: _____

Owner's
Name:_____

Address:_____

City/State/Zip
_____

Telephone:_____E-mail: _____

Pet identification sheet.

> **TWO CATS,**
> **ONE DOG,**
> **AND**
> **TWO TANKS OF**
> **FISH**
> **LIVE IN THIS**
> **HOME.**
> **PLEASE RESCUE IN CASE OF FIRE.**

Window decal to alert firemen and emergency personnel of the presence of pets.

> # HELP!
>
> In the event of an emergency
> Please notify:
>
> ABC Veterinary Hospital
> 1234 Main Street
> Your Town, USA 12345-6789
>
> So that they may care for my unattended pets.

Wallet-sized emergency card.

Sample Text for Reverse Side of Pet Identification Sheet

KEEP YOUR PET SAFE!

Make sure your pet always wears a collar with complete identification tag. Include your pet's name, your name, and your address. We will be glad to help you obtain an identification tag if your pet needs one. Tattoos are more permanent and can be placed in very inconspicuous places.

Always use a leash to take your pet outside.

When riding with your pet in the car, always keep the windows rolled up high enough to prevent him or her from jumping out. But NEVER leave them in a closed car!

During busy times, such as holidays and parties, be extra careful. Strange people and activity in the house can cause your pet to become overexcited and bolt through an open door.

IF YOUR PET IS LOST

Check the neighborhood first. Ask your neighbors if they have seen your pet. Show them the picture on the front.

Let everyone know your pet is missing—neighborhood children, newspaper delivery person, mail carrier, neighbors, joggers, etc. The more people who are aware that your pet is missing, the more chance you will have of finding him or her.

Visit the local animal shelter or humane association to see if your pet has been brought there.

Animal Control Phone #_____

Humane Society Phone #_____

Photocopy the attached flyer with your pet's picture and information. Place the flyers in high traffic areas, such as supermarkets and other area merchants.

Tell us, since often we will get a call based on the rabies tag or our close relations with the animal control teams in our part of the community.

ABC Veterinary Hospital
1234 Main Street
Your Town, USA 12345-6789
(303) 555-1212

Lost Animal Flyer

HELP!

MY PET

IS LOST!

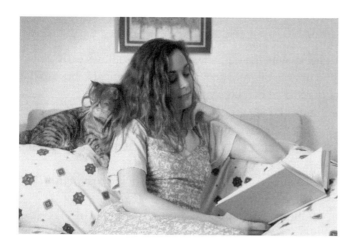

Appendix C

Preferred Client Program

IN 1999, this concept was expanded beyond the traditional uses (high competition, depressed areas, etc.) suggested by Catanzaro and Associates, Inc. It is now more often linked with the reduced vaccination frequency reflex we are seeing from academia (even though we have not seen solid titer protection data in lateral research to support stopping immunization protection). The basic components of the Preferred Client program are presented below. You can find additional details and the *Recovered Patient and Recovered Client Signature Series Monograph* at *www.v-p-c.com.*

Life-Cycle Consultation

Life-cycle consultation is an annual contact with the doctor that is required to "qualify" for "preferred client" status (but each pet is separately qualified). This is not designed as a vaccination or blood drawing event, but rather as a bonding session with the client. The doctor discusses family influences, travel exposure risks, and healthcare concerns during the consultation (the use of the hand-held Heska/PAM/Biolog-type lead-II rhythm cardiac screen in younger animals should lead to better base line data in older animals).

For 12 months, minus one day, after the annual life-cycle consultation, the patient is "qualified" for the balance of the wellness program (many small, economical, fast-in-fast-out visits), including but not limited to:

• Immunization review with outpatient nurse without a doctor's consultation; charged, when administered, at "competitive rates," as compared to the published rates of the community.

- Courtesy dental hygiene checks with the outpatient nurse. This allows early detection of the redness of the gums (pain) and provides an economical access to the teeth cleaning that usually reduces bad breath in companion animals.
- Parasite prevention and control counseling with skilled nurse; if blood or stool samples are required, they are collected and tested at usual practice rates, with the results *always* called back to client; this is done without a doctor's consultation unless results are positive.
- Nutritional advice for dietary needs, again without a doctor's consultation, but with monthly check-ins with the nurse.
- Behavior management, including in-facility source for accessories like scat mats for cats and head collars for dogs, after physiological and medical concerns are eliminated by an outpatient consultation.
- The client is always asked if he/she wants a "doctor's consultation" instead of the nursing appointment, which is "often preferred if [clients] have doctor questions or have not visited with the doctor in the past few months . . . but as a 'preferred client,' it is now their option, not a practice requirement!"
- For twelve months, minus one day, after the annual life-cycle consultation, the client is "qualified" for the communication outreach program, including but not limited to:
  - Periodical newsletters describing new programs and emerging trends in animal wellness and healthcare delivery.
  - Health alerts for specific conditions emerging within the general area or animal population of the community.
  - Specific status reports concerning each animal in the family, their protection level, and special programs which may be accessed.
  - Priority access for doctor's consultations and nursing "hot line" support for the continuing care of the pet.
  - Walk-in privileges whenever the situation is deemed appropriate by the preferred client; no appointment required unless a specific time or specific doctor is desired by the client.

If there is concurrent boarding and/or grooming, preferred clients also will be notified of advanced registration privileges during busy holidays.

Consultant's Observations

- The fact of life is simple; multiple smaller cost visits will cause greater annual value per animal.
- Over 50 percent of all nursing visits will sell something additional.
- Over 23 percent of all boarding or grooming guests need some form of immediate healthcare.
- Smaller tickets reduce ticket shock, make the practice seem more competitive, and better fit tight discretionary spending habits during times of uncertainty or economic stress.
- This program must be tailored to the practice and includes a major effort in

extending the veterinarian's impact by utilizing the paraprofessional staff. In light of this, an on-going in-service training program is *required* to augment the 90-day orientation training plan.

• Over 75 percent of the clients will opt for a doctor's consultation at full price, but it is their option, and they deserve to be seen on time and by the doctor they requested (if any). Never offer a doctor or ask which doctor—if they have a preference, they will tell you!

Consultation vs. Examination

For years we have called the doctor's patient diagnostic exam and client consultation, the sharing of knowledge and skills, by one term, "examination." We were comfortable with this misnomer, even to the extent of hiding the professional effort inside a "vaccination fee"—until the superstore down the street said an "exam" was included with all vaccinations. Panic was a common response, but clarity in services rendered and clearly itemized practice billings were not.

Then the retrospective vaccine panic hit the profession. Some people believed that the vaccinations were "dangerous," and in pursuit of research dollars, they published anecdotal information not substantiated by the traditionally severe drug evaluation criteria. Again, panic was a common response, but clarity in services rendered, and itemized practice billings were not; this time, however, more practices started looking for alternatives to burying everything in the vaccination fee. Clarity of practice billing was not the goal; practitioners were looking for something they could advertise to "beat the competition" and media blitz.

Please stop the insanity. Look at what your practice is doing and start quantifying what your quality of care stands for in the community. Look at a current application of reality and "truth" in performance:

• An animal deserves a annual life-cycle consultation with the doctor. (One dog year is equal to about seven people years, and that is long enough for any living entity to wait for a wellness evaluation!)

• A nurse's wellness examination is done at every entry into the hospital, but the doctor's diagnostic examination is done only when your pet is sick or during the annual life-cycle consultation. This is a critical step in maintaining your pet in a well state, due to the other factors that will be discussed even when your pet appears healthy (as discussed below):

- The consultation will offer discussions about the immunization and protection programs available, as well as when your pet needs to access those services. (It will likely be at a time separate from the consultation, so the cost of the annual life-cycle consultation will seldom be additive, unless the client requests immediate care be rendered.)

- Screening programs for better breath (dentistry), internal body system changes (blood chemistry), and even surveillance of the aging process (radiology and electrocardiograms) will be discussed and scheduled on an as needed basis.

- Families that hike with their pets, take them on vacation, or just live near the fields and woods may need additional protection; that is also discussed and planned during the doctor's consultation.

- Fleas and ticks, as well as some internal parasites, can be deterred from attacking your pet. These alternatives will be discussed during the consultation, and options will be provided for the client's consideration.

As you can see, most of the consultation elements above require (1) participative listening, (2) assessment of internal, external, or environmental dangers, and (3) subsequent client communications. If your practice takes time to listen to clients, healthcare access is increased in most A and B clients, and often even in the C clients. If the practice tries to do all of the above with only doctors, you cannot afford the effort. If you use an outpatient nursing program concurrent with high density scheduling, clients will begin to equate veterinary healthcare with other healthcare delivery models. Human outpatient clinics use three to five examination rooms per doctor, and dentists use four to eight chairs per doctor. Clients will start to understand that "technicians" are really nurses, with exceptional skills and knowledge about companion animals and, generally, with far greater abilities and capabilities than most of their human medicine counterparts.

So, undifferentiated examination by habit, or clarity in quality with the consultation; the choice is yours today. With failure to change, you will either lose the option or become an "old timer"; neither role will attract the quality client to your practice. Slow death is painful . . . and for the want of a horseshoe nail, the war was lost!

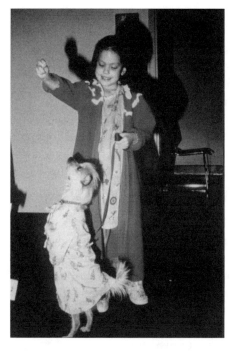

Courtesy of Children's and Delta Society.

Appendix D

Behavior Management: A New Continuing Education Experience

Education is only a ladder to gather fruit from the tree of knowledge, not the fruit itself.
—Anonymous

THE IDEAS are many, the interest is high. Stewards of animals want well-behaved family members. In fact, multiple surveys have shown that 90 percent of owners want some form of behavior management assistance with a pet. Behavior management is a veterinarian's duty (it usually starts with house training), to ensure a proper family fit for the pet. Obedience training is not behavior management, and I am not advocating veterinarians get into obedience training. Behavior management is a lifestyle situation that practice staff members need to become involved in to extend animal lives and improve the quality of family support for the animal the family share its life with; it is also a client-bonding activity that makes practice fun again.

Yet practices continue to "push" vaccinations for diseases that are seldom, if ever, seen, and they worry about feed store sales competition, rather than meeting their clients' needs. Practices send thousands of reminders for distemper vaccinations, but seldom see a case; they send no reminders for behavior, yet they see multiple cases each day. Even to the most casual observer, there is something wrong with this picture. This is called "wearing blinders" in some situations, but more often, it is just a *lost opportunity* to become indispensable within a community to your clients (not to mention the loss in net income that occurs when this need for behavior management is ignored).

During recent practice consultations, as we discussed the merits of behavior management as an income center, it became clear that some practices that we support could not make the leap of faith from theory to reality. They knew a few resources, from pamphlets to the Promise head collar, and they knew that their clients needed the service, but they had not convinced themselves that they could charge for it. Some did not know the current theory or had been confused by brief articles in the literature that seemed disjointed. How to deliver behavior management as a meaningful service, specifically a fee-for-service, needed to be based upon confidence of success and methodologies of marketing. It became evident that progressive practice management, marketing, and promotion techniques *needed* to be integrated into the academic pursuit of knowledge. We choose a seminar, "Behavior Management as an Income Center," as our first attempt!

Methodology

The primary subject matter experts were Daniel Q. Estep and Suzanne Hetts, both certified animal behaviorists (see appendix E). The business management and marketing vignettes were done by myself, and the client and staff marketing communication methods were done by L. Susan Bochatey, of Catanzaro and Associates, Inc., on the last day of the 20-hour seminar. The vignettes were called "Mini–Management Moments" and were provided once mid-morning and once mid-afternoon on the first two days of the course. On the last day, it was all tied together by providing break-out sessions where the participants actually started to integrate the behavior management ideas into their annual marketing plans. This first seminar was centered on behavior problem prevention, and there is a subsequent seminar in the planning to deal with resolving existing behavior problems. In 2000, AAHA teamed up with Dan and Suzanne to repeat these programs.

The training approach taken by this team was structured to be similar to that encountered in veterinary school. The first section was the basic sciences, the principles and systems that must be understood before application can be attempted. The second phase was the clinical years, where applications were made to real life experiences, but still within the context of the education process. The third phase was the reality of practice, where the basic sciences and clinical years must be integrated into practice with economics, people, programs, staff, clients, associate veterinarians, and community mores as mediating factors. Most every participant left wanting to know more about problem resolution. They were ready to attend the next seminar. This is the mark of a *great* continuing education experience. Any practice can simulate this same environment by training their trainers at regional continuing education conferences, using the new references offered by AAHA, or even attending seminars like the one outlined above, then making the time for a practice-specific, practical, in-service seminar.

Another way to look at this new method of training, combining the technical skills with management, marketing, and business alternatives, is to view the experience in light of some of the comments received in the seminar evaluations:

Excellent—a real effort was made to give us information we could take home ... so many handouts! It seemed every good idea was followed by a handout.

I was exposed to a whole new way of thinking.

Very good plan of action. Good combination of practical information combined with management and marketing. Good pace.

Liked (loved) concept of behavior prevention with animal behavior problems as well as seeing the staff as clients.

Excellent flow and content—it was very helpful to know how to integrate these ideas into our practice.

Some Key Ideas

It is not nice to tease the reader, so the following is a look at one segment of the technical aspects of behavior management, first impressions:

- When a dog pulls an owner through the front door, behavior management is needed. A staff that is "tuned in on behavior management" will address this situation *before* the client enters the examination room, with something as simple as one of the new "head collars" that provide for almost immediate "power steering" and control of the animal.
- When a new puppy is presented, house training assistance *must* be provided, if the practice believes in behavior management. If this courtesy service appears on the invoice as a "$20 behavior management consultation" and is given as a courtesy, the tone *and the price* have been set for further encounters.
- The Behavior Management "New Pet" Owners Orientation, held outside for puppies and inside for kittens after Saturday appointments and in nice weather, is offered as a one-time "courtesy session." It is offered to all humane society adoptions, pet store purchases, and new vaccination clients. It is a staff time to discuss the basics, from socialization, to handling, to grooming, to wellness care.

The above three ideas are obvious. The family fit, animal socialization, and basic behavior management services can be offered by even the most neophyte of staff members, if properly trained. While problem prevention is easy, in some of the more advanced behavior problems, referral is needed. The nice thing about behavior problems is that many of the referral cases can be done by telephone. The choice to participate is an individual commitment, and the market is there.

The ability to meet the needs of the community is based in the practice philosophy. Whether your practice wants to gather this "fruit" or let it lie and rot is now up to you, but remember, over five million animals a year are euthanized because of behavior problems. Save lives or contribute to this number, the choice is yours.

The Behavior Management as an Income Center agenda is provided below:

      Gathering and Introductions

      Your Role in Behavior Counseling

      Behavior Development of Puppies and Kittens

      Puppy Classes

      MINI-MANAGEMENT MOMENT #1 (puppy clubs)

      Pet Selection

      MINI-MANAGEMENT MOMENT #2 (existing resources)

      Litter box "Training" for Kittens

      Crates and Confinement

      MINI-MANAGEMENT MOMENT #3 (resale perspectives)

      House training Puppies

      Destructive Behaviors

      Puppy and Kitten Aggressive Behaviors

      Introduction of Puppies and Kittens to Resident Animals

      MINI-MANAGEMENT MOMENT #4 (vaccination sequence alternatives)

      Puppies, Kittens, and Kids

      Owner Communication Skills

      PRACTICE MANAGEMENT and MARKETING PLAN

      Graduation

Mini-Management Moments

#1 Implementation of Puppy Clubs and Kitten Carrier Classes

The Puppy Club can be different from the traditional Puppy Kindergarten course. While the Puppy Kindergarten is usually a trainer's introductory program offered as a fee-for-instruction service, the Puppy Club is more social and is designed for a technician to help bond clients to the practice, so it is usually a "courtesy service" offered to puppy owners. A fee-for-service program carries with it a liability and an implied contract agreement, while a social program with no fee reduces the liability and implied contract concerns. The total integrated package is offered as a way to help practices understand that it is not a single service or a set program: it is a process of bonding a client to the practice, of meeting the needs of the owner (e.g., 90 percent of new owners desire assistance with behavior management of their pet), and of expanding the professional image of the practice team. It is an opportunity to be a leader in your community.

The Puppy Club has been done in many formats, but the most exciting is the one conducted by the veterinary practice's paraprofessional team. It is an opportunity for the staff to talk to clients in the evening, 60 minutes maximum since the puppies have a 15 minute maximum tolerance, and help them become better stewards of their companion animals. The Kitten Carrier Class is an extension of this concept, since we want the owners of all critters to bond to the practice with this "value added" service. Please keep the kittens and puppies on different nights.

The classes are formatted around the expertise of your staff. The technician discusses common postneonatal questions, nutrition, hygiene, and wellness issues. Socialization is simply getting the animals used to coming to the practice without always receiving an injection. The reasons this concept requires multiple visits, other than the familiarity associated with smelling other animals, being handled by other people, and traveling often by car without pain, include the following:

- It is an opportunity to help the owners deal with feet (nails), ears (plucking and cleaning), tails (anals), teeth (brushing), and other anatomically awkward appendages.
- It is the time to discuss parasites (prevention as well as control), nutrition (diets and treats), and behavior management (e.g., Gentle Leader—Promise head collar).
- In puppies, if behavior management includes floor work by group, try to keep the class members (puppies) within five weeks of age of each other. Again, the simplest of concepts are only used for 10–15 minutes at a time, then the puppies are allowed to rest while other subjects are discussed with the owners.

The attendance has no requirements, for the pet or the owner. There are no strings attached. It is a low investment for a practice (utilities, two hours of technician time, and initial refreshments). If the social period really takes off, the participants may even offer to bring refreshments. Let them feel needed! If at some point in the process, clients want to know more about behavior specifically for their pet, they can be referred to either the practice appointment schedule or an area behavior specialist.

The technician's fee approximates the practice office call, about $20 for 20 minutes, with weekly review appointments until the behavior has been modified. Some progressive practices are now booking 55 technician behavior management appointments per month. Please see the sample forms and invitation cards provided for initial implementation ideas for your practice.

#2 Implementation of Existing Resources

You don't need to reinvent the wheel! The AVMA has produced beautiful color brochures (about $15.00 per 100). You need to invent a delivery system in your community! The Delta Society (206/226-7357) has the starting point. The Delta Society is an international clearinghouse of human-animal bond programs, from assistance animals to pet libraries in schools. Your practice may know what is needed, or you may want to look at existing resources for ideas. Either way, don't start from scratch. Learn from those who have gone before. Please review the resources provided.

Some have started their "Pets by Prescription Program" (a Delta Society term) in the school, by doing in-service orientations to teachers and counselors using the historical success stories from Delta Society (stuttering children, insecurities, etc.). Others have offered third-party, not-for-fee assistance to pet stores and humane societies in the area, to assist their clients in getting the right pet for the family (e.g., Bassets are cute, but are not for joggers). The third-party assistance to pet stores relieves the store from the liability perception imparted by clerks who recommend an animal just "to get rid of it from inventory."

The current literature carries ideas from Dr. Ron Whitford on how he set his wife up in a nonprofit corporation (cost about $50,000, including facility) specifically to place well puppies and kittens in the community. In addition to the adoption fee, his wife's corporation requires that the animals receive all their care from her husband's clinic. They are now shipping about 50 percent of the Tennessee animals to New York for placement (another fee for service from the nonprofit corporation). The AVMA Trust sees excessive liability with this concept.

Again, the pet selection assistance is usually a courtesy service, based on the concept that happy clients will return to the practice for pet healthcare. It starts the bonding even *before* the pet enters the family.

#3 Implementation of Retail Sales Resources

Very seldom does any practice consider behavior management a retail sales opportunity—thank goodness. Behavior management is as close to a pure service as is surgical time for a doctor. There are some retail sales associated with behavior management, but they must be kept in perspective.

Crates are a very helpful aid when a pet is sent home on restricted activity. They are also very helpful when introducing a new animal to a resident animal. Some practices move enough crates through their facilities to be able to price them lower than the community discount stores (Wal-Mart, PetsMart, etc.), but an approximately equal price is an appropriate target. This retail service is especially important when instructing clients how to size crates and how to use them for behavior or healthcare management.

Leashes and collars are another resale line that goes underutilized. Some practices make receptionists accountable for the display and stocking by giving them a cut of the action. You would be surprised how displays improve and sales increase. A specialized offering like the Promise or Gentle Leader head collar needs to be seen as only part of a training management system. The head collar is designed to use only instinctive pressures (why is the only animal we train by choking "man's best friend"?) and can get a client to return to the practice frequently. As such, the head collar should be retailed for only slightly over cost (in quantity, they are not available for less than $13.00 per system, so a $15.00 resale would be adequate. The head collar alone is less than $9.00, so resale could be only $11.00). The money is made on the subsequent training session—*or*—on the now well-behaved patient.

One-stop shopping is needed in many communities, and in others it is not needed. The choice is a strategic practice concern. It is my opinion that a companion animal practice should *never* replace outpatient exam space with retail space. It can't produce net income as well as professional healthcare delivery. Better use of waiting room or reception space is a different issue.

#4 Implementation with Vaccination Programs

With a full exam with every puppy or kitten vaccination, fees for a rabies-distemper visit are approaching $100; meanwhile the newspaper advertises multiple sources for getting a $20 rabies-distemper alternative. In this situation, where do you *expect* the average uninformed pet owner to go? As an alternative puppy/kitten program:

• First vaccination, doctor's consultation and house-training information (offer to send home numbered videotape for family viewing) (qualifies client/patient for puppy club).
• Second vaccination, technician exam and socialization information (offer to send home numbered videotape for family viewing) (requalifies client/patient for puppy club).
• Third vaccination, doctor's consultation and family-fit information (offer to send home numbered videotape for family viewing) (requalifies client/patient for puppy club).

• Behavior management assistance is provided by the technician *after* the doctor leaves the exam room. This sets the tone for later efforts in dental, nutrition, and parasite control counseling.
• Numbered videotapes (AVLS/PETCOM, PROMISE) help ensure tracking; tape is not a rental, just a loaner.
• Puppy club should be made available through the first six months of age (to the neutering decision, OHE or castration).
• The invoice should specifically state the behavior counseling effort: house training, socialization, family fit, or whatever was conducted.

Some practices provide a pet-specific $5.00 pet population control credit (deducted from the standard OHE/castration fee) with each vaccination, redeemable with appointments made between five and six months of age. This not only builds the appropriate expectations within the client's mind, it also gives the impression of a preferred client benefit and brings the surgery into a more competitive price range. Build and deliver the program that provides "added value" for clients. Make them feel special!

Suggested Indications for a Behavior Medical Workup

Problems Indicating Need for Workup	Problems for Which No Workup Is Routinely Done
Canine Behavior	
Aggression; growling, snapping, snarling; fighting	Begging
Coprophagy	Car chasing
Destructive digging	Charging
Destructive chewing	Crotch sniffing
Escaping	Dislikes the vet/groomer
Excessive licking	Disobedient
Excessive vocalization barking, howling, whining	Jumping up
Excitatory urination	Killing animals (predatory)
Fearful of objects	Leash pulling
Fearful of other dogs	Possessive
Fearful of people	Puppy biting
Garbage eating	Up on furniture
House soiling	
Hyperactive	
Lack of response to name	
Motion sickness	
Mounting	
Obsessive compulsive behavior	
Refuses grooming	
Rolling in filth	
Self-mutilation	
Shyness	
Stealing food	
Submissive urination	
Toilet drinking	
Urine marking	

Problems Indicating Need for Workup	Problems for Which No Workup Is Routinely Done
Feline Behavior	
Aggression (including biting)	Aloof/independent
Destructive to household	Climbing curtains
Excessive grooming	Excessive kneading and
Excessive vocalization	suckling
Fearful	Roaming
Fighting	Up on counters
Finicky	
Hissing	
Hyperactive	
Inappropriate elimination	
Obsessive compulsive	
Destructive scratching	
Stalks owner	

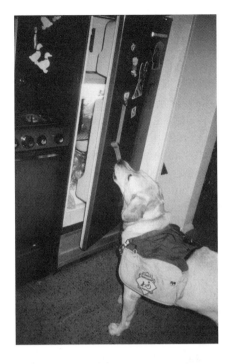

Courtesy of Nancy McKenna
and Delta Society.

Appendix E

Behavior Trainers: Professional Behavior Management Help

AUTHOR'S NOTE: This appendix provides a few sample ideas for a letter/brochure for veterinary practice clients. With training and continuing education, most veterinary practices can provide the initial behavior management assistance to clients, but as in first aid care, the practice must know when to refer to a specialist. When a physiological basis has been ruled out, and the staff has tried, do not hesitate to call for assistance. There needs to be a behaviorist on-call to your practice just as there is an orthopedic surgeon or an internal medicine specialist.

Special recognition for these contributions goes to Daniel O. Estep, Ph.D., and Suzanne Hetts, Ph.D., Animal Behavior Associates, Inc., 4994 S. Independence Way, Littleton, CO 80123, (303) 932-9095.

A Veterinary Practice Guide to Finding Professional Help for Animal Behavior Problems

Knowing who to turn to when your companion animal is misbehaving can be a confusing process. Well-meaning people may have already given you suggestions which are at odds with each other, and you don't know who to believe. People who work with animal behavior problems are not regulated by any government agency and may have very different types of qualifications. You need to know what questions to ask to evaluate their training. This brochure provides you with information about various types of animal-related professionals, how they are trained, and what professional credentials to look for, in order to find the person who best meets your needs.

The volunteers who staff behavior help lines at humane societies, like the Denver Dumb Friends League, have completed an extensive training program taught by the on-staff certified applied animal behaviorist. The training program includes both lecture and supervised experience.

Veterinarians

Clients know that their first call for a pet that is having a problem should always be to their regular veterinarian. Urinary tract infections, hormone imbalances, neurological conditions, orthopedic problems, or dental disease are just a few examples of medical problems which can affect behavior and cause problems such as house soiling or aggression. The veterinarian must do the physical examination and diagnostic screening before any form of behavior management is considered.

A great deal of variation exists in how much training in animal behavior veterinarians receive in school. Some receive very little, while others have taken advantage of clinical behavioral elective courses or have even obtained postgraduate degrees in a behavioral science. In 1995, it became possible for veterinarians to become Board Certified in Behavior by the AVMA's Behavior College. Ask your veterinarian what kind of specific training in animal behavior she/he has received. Most veterinarians readily recognize the advantage of referring behavior cases to a behavioral specialist, just as they would refer complicated cardiology or cancer cases to medical or surgical specialists.

Certified Applied Animal Behaviorists

Perhaps the greatest confusion in finding professional help for your pet's behavior problem lies in the distinction between animal trainers and animal behaviorists. People who have worked with or trained animals for many years are not animal behaviorists unless they have specialized academic training.

Animal behavior is a specialized field of scientific study, as are clinical psychology, social work, and veterinary medicine. In order to become an applied animal behaviorist, an individual must have specialized training not only in the broad field of animal behavior, but also in that part of behavior which relates to behavior problems in companion animals. In 1991, professional certification for applied animal behaviorists became available from the Animal Behavior Society (ABS), which is the primary professional organization for the study of animal behavior in the United States

Certification indicates that the behaviorist is academically trained, has experience in the field, and meets the ethical standards of the ABS. To become certified, behaviorists must document their training, provide letters of referral from other ABS members, and submit three case studies for review by the Board of Certification. You should ask the animal behaviorist what graduate degree he/she has (M.S. or Ph.D.), in what field (a behavioral science such as animal psychology or ethology), and if he/she is certified.

Behavior Consultants with Graduate Degrees

Graduate degree programs which provide the necessary training for applied animal behavior consulting are in a behavioral science (not chemistry or geology for example), should include animal learning theory and ethology (understanding how to observe and interpret behavior), and should involve learning how to apply this information to behavior problems in companion animals. Ask consultants what graduate degree they have (M.S. or Ph.D), in what field, what courses they took, how they obtained their applied experience, and if they are eligible for certification.

Animal Trainers

Most animal trainers are self-taught; obedience training is not a standard science, and there are many schools of thought. Some may have apprenticed under another trainer and/or attended various training seminars. Animal trainers typically are not trained in the study of animal behavior, and many use punishment (e.g., choke collars, shock collars, etc.). Trainers are usually available for birds, horses, and dogs, but not often for cats (cat owners will say they are too smart to be trained, but the simple fact is that there is not a lot of money in becoming a cat trainer). Good animal trainers are knowledgeable about many different types of training methods and use techniques which neither the animal nor the owner find consistently unpleasant.

Good training methods should focus primarily on reinforcing good behavior and should use punishment sparingly, appropriately, and humanely. Using choke chains to lift dogs off the ground and "string them up" is *not* appropriate or humane; nor is excessive use of force with whips or other devices with horses.

Dog obedience classes are an excellent way to develop a good relationship with your dog and to gain more control over him by teaching him to respond reliably to specific commands. However, resolving behavior problems such as house soiling, barking, aggression, or separation anxiety requires more than teaching your dog commands. Specific behavior modification techniques must also be used. Some animal trainers also offer behavior consulting services.

Ask trainers what type of methods they use, how they were trained, and if they will allow you to observe their classes. If you observe techniques which you are not comfortable with, find another trainer. Dog obedience instructors can be endorsed by the National Association of Dog Obedience Instructors (NADOI). Endorsement indicates that an instructor has been approved by his/her peers and uses humane methods of training. If the trainer is endorsed by another organization, ask what the criteria for endorsement are.

Things to Watch for and Avoid

- Anyone who guarantees their work. Animals are living beings, not dishwashers with warranties. Qualified behaviorists and trainers will always do their best for you, but they cannot guarantee outcomes because animals have minds of their own and can never be completely controlled by humans.
- People whose *primary* methods or style focus on punishment. If their first recommendations involve choking, hitting, or slapping the animal, confinement, or isolation, they have little or no understanding of animal behavior.
- People who misrepresent their qualifications. People who call themselves animal behaviorists, even though they are not trained in animal behavior.
- People who want to take the animal and train it for you. Most behavior problems are a result of interactions between the animal, the owner, and the environment. Giving the animal to someone else to "fix" the problem is rarely successful because these three elements are not addressed. Owners need to work with the animal in the home environment.

If you are committed to working with your pet, and find qualified people to help you, the chances of successfully resolving many problem behaviors are great.

Resources

1. Delta Society (800-869-6898), 289 Perimeter Road East, Renton, WA 98055-1329.
2. Latham Letter, Latham Plaza Building, 1826 Clement Avenue, Alameda, CA 94501.
3. CENSHARE, 611 Bencar St., SE, University of Minnesota, Minneapolis, MN 55455.

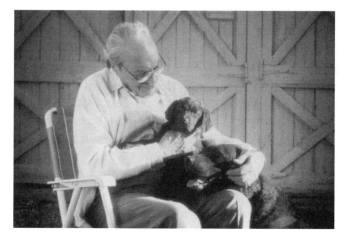

Appendix F

The Art of Communication with Dogs

Introduction

DOGS AND humans are blessed with the gift of being "best friends." This did not come about by accident. We both belong to the group of animals known as pack animals. As pack animals we share certain things in common which are dictated by our need for social interaction. We must have order and routine in our lives or we become cranky. Out of our basic understanding of a hierarchical structure comes the need to have an authority figure in our lives or we become the "boss." We not only want, but need discipline in our lives. The success or failure of our ability to attain these things lies in the success of our communication skills.

Both humans and dogs use the same two elements to have successful communication skills: body language—what you do, often unconsciously, with your facial expressions, posture, arms, and legs; and paralanguage—the sounds that come out of your throat, that make words, that have meaning.

Common Body Language

• *Self-confidence.* Standing erect and using direct eye contact.
• *"I'm more important than you are."* Standing erect with hands at hips or arms crossed, often with the neck arched tall and "looking down the nose" at the other party. We even seem to take a deep breath to puff ourselves up to be bigger. (In addition to this, dogs will tip their ears forward and when they feel especially threatened, they will bristle their fur and sometimes show their teeth.)

- *Insecurity/uneasiness.* Slumping and looking away.
- *Fear or contrition.* Bowing down, pulling head into shoulders, looking down. (In addition, dogs roll their ears back and tuck their tails under their belly.)
- *Extreme fear.* Dropping to the ground or rolling over on their back. Body will remain stiff (in contrast to a request for a belly rub, when the body is very relaxed). Possible urination or anal gland release (to expose scent).
- *"Let's play."* Head cocks sideways or head bows and eyes shift to the top of the head; the whole body may squirm with anticipation.

Common Paralanguage

- *Nurturing or soft controlling sounds.* Cooing or "baby talk."
- *"Let's play"/"We're 'equal'"/"We're just having fun."* High pitched "yip, yip, yip" sound. *Palaver* (idle chatter or beguiling talk between persons of different levels; often used to cajole or persuade with deliberate flattery). Examples: "Good dog!" "Atta boy!" "Good job!" "Better!" "That's the way!"
- *Warning.* Low guttural "growl" sound. Examples: "No-o-o!" "Sha-a-me!" "Ba-a-ad Dog!" "Mi-i-ine!" "Leave it!"
- *Alert/danger.* Sharp "bark" sound. Examples: "Out!" "Off!" "No!" "Quiet!" "Stop!" (Please note: These are all *one-word, one-syllable, one-time* sounds. To repeat the sound as in "No, no, no!" or "Stop it, stop it!" will sound more like "Yip, yip, yip!" This is *faulty paralanguage* because the dog will interpret this as the "Let's play" sound. Along this same line, *all commands should be given only once* (i.e., "Sit!"). "Sit . . . sit . . . sit" sounds more like "Get up and play, play, play!"

Canine Behavior Management Begins with the ABC's

"Best friend" relationships need not be difficult or complicated if you simply stick to the basics, play fair, and stay consistent. It's easy to build a relationship with your dog if you, the more intelligent part of the team, will consider what is natural for the dog:

- Dogs (like humans) are pack animals by nature and must have another warm being in their lives. They adapt well to the recognized social order of the pack.
- *Alpha.* Dogs understand and respect the authority figure in their lives. If no one else is perceived as the "boss," the dog will appoint himself as alpha (or head of the pack).
- *Basic survival needs.* The two most basic survival needs for dogs are not the people in their lives. They are simply *food and shelter.* Because of their importance, it is quite easy to apply "rules" to these things to help establish yourself as head of the pack.
- *Communication.* As members of a pack, dogs understand and use communication skills that are very similar to our human forms of communication. Dog and man are more alike in this regard than any other species. Perhaps this is why we are so naturally suited to be best friends.

- *Discipline.* Dogs can live well within the system of the pack because they respect the "pecking order" within the pack. Each member knows his place within the chain of command, and all members expect and accept some form of discipline if they step out of line.
- *Environmental control.* Dogs understand boundary lines or "turf." (They mark theirs with urine, we mark ours with walls, doors, fences, gates, and invisible property lines.) Proper environmental control is basic to teaching your dog the rules within the pack.
- In addition, *best friends* never embarrass or take advantage of each other.

The Golden Rule seems to say it best.

The Ground Rules of Pet Training

- Prevention is easier than a cure. If an animal is exposed to the right things at the right stages in his life, it does make a difference!
- Pets learn by trial and error.
- We use the *same methods* to teach an animal to *do* something as we do to teach him *not to do* other things.
- There is more than one way to train an animal. If the method we choose does not seem to be working, we simply go back to the drawing board until we find the animal's "hot button."
- There are no quick fixes. Trying new methods one time will not solve a problem.
- Animals establish new habit patterns by repetitions of behavior. In most cases, it takes *six weeks* to undo a naughty behavior! (That is, six weeks of never letting the behavior occur! If the pet slips up and successfully carries out the behavior during the modification time frame, the behavior actually becomes an intermittent reward and will make the behavior worse than it was before!)
- Use methods that involve both positive and negative rewards.
- The three phases of training are
  - *Place.* Place the animal in a position where he can't make a mistake. Limit his choices.
  - *Practice.* By using repetition to our advantage, the pet will establish new habit patterns of behavior.
  - *Test.* Does the pet clearly *understand* what his proper behavior should be? You won't know unless you set up a few "controlled distractions." Test his knowledge skills and be prepared to communicate with some well-timed discipline.
- Animal training is not difficult if a person knows how to effectively use the tools of consistency, environmental control, and good communication and disciplinary skills.

Teaching Your Puppy to "Come" and "Sit" at Your Feet

The three most important things you will ever teach your puppy are to (a) *Trust* you, (b) *Come* when you call, and (c) *Sit* quietly at your feet. The sooner you begin to make these exercises a natural part of your relationship, the better. Make use of your puppy's instinctive desire to win your approval and make use of his natural curiosity. Use your puppy's name frequently. Always associate his name with praise and reward. If you call him by name and then punish him it won't be long before he's running away from you rather than coming to you. Make *his name* and *"come"* the two most rewarding words he'll ever know.

Begin by carrying your puppy to a new (distraction free) area. Place him on the ground, call his name and say "Come" as you walk away. Being a pack animal, your puppy will most likely choose not to be left behind. After he follows a few steps, *drop down to his level* and let him catch up with you. When he comes all the way to you, *lift his head and scoop his bottom into a sit.* (Do not get into the habit of reaching for your puppy before he comes all the way to you! He will *think* this is a game and will learn to play "keep away" by staying just out of range.)

Continue to pet and praise your puppy as you *look him in the eye. A puppy who learns there is reward for sitting at a person's feet* when he's called will not jump on people later! If your puppy begins to lose interest in this new game, run away from him. This will usually activate the "chase instinct." Reward him with a food treat *before* you help him into a sit position. Make the reward something your puppy really likes (i.e., cheese, liver treats, hot dogs).

It may be necessary to become a good actor. Touch and talk to the grass and imaginary bugs in a very excited voice. Curiosity will usually win out, and your puppy will come to see what excitement he's missing.

After a few days of enthusiastic responses to "come," begin to play "come games" with your puppy. Hide-and-seek games are fun as long as you hide in relatively simple places. Don't try to trick your puppy. The object of this game is to build your puppy's confidence. *You* become *the prize* for a job well done. Always reward your puppy on his level as you help him into a sit.

Another good way to practice "come" and exercise a puppy at the same time is to teach him to come back and forth between two or more people. Practice this exercise on leash just in case you need a check cord. You will let the leash drag behind your puppy. Take your puppy and a friend to a safe open field. Have your friend squat down to visit with your puppy. Then turn the puppy so he can watch you leave. Turn your back on your puppy and run several steps away. Turn around to face your puppy, squat down, and call him to you. Use his name followed by the command, "Come." When he arrives at your feet, gently lift his head and scoop his bottom into a sit. After praising profusely, turn the puppy around so he can see his new friend *jump up,* run *straight* away, turn, squat, and invite him to come. Have your friend reward your puppy with a treat, lift his head, and tuck him into a sit. Repeat. Your puppy will be running back and forth as the distance increases. In the event that your puppy is hesitant to leave your side to go to your friend, take the leash *and run with your puppy.* Once your puppy understands what is expected and has focused his attention on your friend, drop the leash and allow him complete the trip on his own.

Teaching Your Puppy to "Sit" and "Wait"

Teaching your puppy to "sit" on command is as easy as getting his attention and getting him to *look up*. You'll understand what I mean if you will get down on your hands and knees. Try to drink out of a paper cup without spilling a drop. Keep your hands on the floor. After you have lifted your chin as high as you can go, you'll find yourself "sitting" to avoid getting wet. A young puppy is very clumsy and can not look up without sitting down. It's that simple!

Use treats that are sure to get your puppy's attention (i.e., liver treats, cheese bits, hot dog slices). Show the treat to your puppy at his *nose level*. When he has fixed his attention on the treat, walk backwards a few steps and encourage him *to follow the treat*. While his nose is still glued to the treat, say his name and the command, "Sit." Take a step toward your puppy and lift the treat slightly above his head. This should cause him to flop into a sit. Reward him immediately! *If he tries to jump up,* you are probably holding the treat too high up. Lower the treat to nose level and take another step into your puppy as you repeat the command to "sit." You may find it helpful to practice this on leash the first few tries. Let the reward come from your *right hand*. Obedience trained dogs respond to a right-hand signal which moves from the handler's hip to his shoulder in a "palm up" fashion.

After a few successful responses on *the first command* to "sit," begin to teach your puppy to "wait" or "stay" for a few seconds before receiving his reward. Rotate your hand over and spread your fingers wide to form a "wall" directly in front of your puppy's eyes. Use the leash to keep a mild upward pull on the back of your puppy's head. This will encourage him to keep his head up and his bottom down. Two seconds is long enough to wait in the beginning. As your puppy grows steadier, begin to stand taller and add distance between the hand holding the treat and the tip of your dog's nose. If your puppy starts to jump for the treat, you are probably progressing too fast. Repeat the "sit . . . wait" command and move the "wall" back to nose level. A gentle upward snap with the collar and leash will serve as a reminder to keep his head up. Just for fun, watch your dog get up from a sit position. Balance requires him to lower his head and shift his weight forward before standing. If he keeps his *head up, his bottom will stay down.*

Clicker Training

Clicker training is designed to help your dog learn *how* to learn. It quickly teaches him to *listen* for a sound, to *look* to you for directions, to *respond* in an appropriate manner, and to *receive a reward* for a job well done.

When you make the "click" sound, it is very important to make the sound **only once.** The same is true when you give commands later on. To issue the command more than once will encourage your dog to "stall" or to learn to turn a deaf ear to your commands. Don't get in the habit of training him to bad habits. When you begin, be sure to stand an arm's distance away so the sound is not so loud that it frightens your dog. Hold the clicker in your *left* hand and the treat in your *right* hand. Since obedience hand signals are given with the right hand, this naturally encourages your dog to look for your right hand.

Treats should be really special and should be broken into small pieces. Be sure to offer the treat at the level of the dog's nose to prevent him from jumping. If he does not already take treats gently from your hand, teach him to do so *before* you start clicker training. (Wrap your fingers completely around the treat. If your dog snaps for the treat, give him what he wanted, but give him *more than* he bargained for. Push your entire hand into his mouth as you bark, "No!" He will probably gag slightly. Offer the treat again and command, "Easy." If he licks for the treat, gently slide it toward the end of your fingertips and place it into his mouth. Praise him lavishly with "Good Dog!")

Let's get started.

Stage 1: Click—Reward

Click the clicker once. Reward your dog with a treat *immediately.* Timing is very important. If you wait for a response, you have waited too long. After about three click-reward sequences, your dog will begin to respond to the sound. Wait five minutes and begin again. This time, click and pause. The *instant* the dog indicates he heard something (he does not have to look at you, he only has to flick an ear or an eyebrow to indicate he heard), *place* the treat in his mouth and *praise.* (Do not call him to you.) Go to his other side and repeat the process. When he starts to turn in the direction of your hand, stand behind him. If he will turn completely around to find the sound, you are ready to move on to Stage 2. *Note:* The key to this stage is surprise. It may be hard to get your dog to ignore you once he realizes you have a pocketful of treats. Be patient. Wait until he is not watching before clicking the clicker again.

Stage 2: Name—Click—Reward

You should now be four to six feet away from your dog. Quietly say his name, click the clicker, and squat down to meet him on his level. Place the food directly into your dog's mouth. He should only have to move a few feet in your direction before getting his treat. When he consistently comes running across the room, go to Stage 3.

Stage 3: Name—Click—"Come"—Reward

You should spend *three* days at Stage 3. At this stage, gradually add distance and be creative! Work indoors and outside. Play hide and seek as you duck behind a door or behind a bush. This simple exercise teaches your dog to use reasoning skills to find you. Notice that your dog is now doing a *series* of things before he receives his reward. You should still squat down to meet him on his level. Be *generous* with verbal and physical rewards! "Come" will soon become his favorite game.

Stage 4: Name—Click—"Come"—"Sit"—Reward

This stage begins the same as Stage 3 with two exceptions: When your dog gets within two feet of you, *stand* and go to meet him. As you greet your dog, tell him to sit.

Lift his head by "gluing" the treat to his nose and raising your hand slightly as you step into him. (Keep your palm up. In the future, this gesture will become the hand signal to sit.) This action should cause him to lift his head. If his chin goes up, his center of gravity shifts and his bottom should go down. (You may need to assist by pulling the leash up with your left hand.) If he jumps up, you are probably holding the treat too high. Tap him lightly on the nose with the back of your hand. At the same time, bark, "No!" Step into him and repeat the "sit" command. If necessary, help him into a sit and *praise* to be sure he understands that "sit" is the desired behavior.

After a full week at Stage 4, begin to alternate between food rewards and praise-only rewards in an attempt to wean your dog from food rewards altogether. *After another week,* begin to alternate the use of the clicker with just the "come" command. In time, your dog should be very eager to respond to the command to come by spinning on a dime and running to sit at your feet.

Clicker training may also be an effective tool to use to defuse a potentially stressful situation for your dog. (That is, thunderstorms, fear of the leash, or signs of impending aggression. *Note:* This will not stop aggression that has already begun, but it may redirect your dog's attention and therefore prevent a situation from starting.)

To teach a show dog to "bait" for the conformation ring the easy way, *clicker train* him.

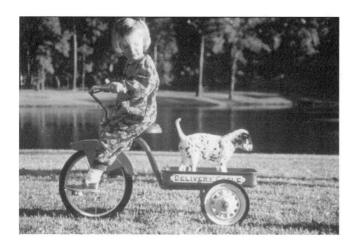

Appendix G

For the New Puppy Owner

THE MATERIAL presented in this appendix represents a series of handouts for new and prospective dog owners and includes an outline of the material covered in a "puppy class."

So You Want a Dog? Some Things for Prospective Dog Owners to Think About

Bringing a dog into your home is a wonderful experience, but it is also a serious responsibility. Below are some questions for you and your family members to ask yourselves about your own needs and expectations of the dog that will help you pick out the pet best suited to you. Try to be as realistic and honest as possible in answering these questions.

1. Why do you want a dog?

What do you expect the dog to do? Will she just be a companion for you? Will she be a companion for your children? Do you want a dog you can jog or hike with? A dog to hunt with? A watch dog or a guard dog? A working dog like a herding dog? A show dog? Do you want the dog to serve several roles? (Note

---

Special Recognition for these contributions goes to Daniel O. Estep, Ph.D., and Suzanne Hetts, Ph.D., Animal Behavior Associates, Inc., 4994 S. Independence Way, Littleton, CO 80123, (303) 932-9095.

that some roles may not be compatible: A good guard dog may not be good around your children.) Different breeds or individuals within a breed may be better suited to some roles than to others.

2. What's your family like now? What do you expect it to be in 5 to 10 years?

Are you single, married, or married with children; do you have older relatives in the home? Are you single now but expect to start a family soon? Your choice of pet should take into account not only your present family status but also your expected future status. A dog chosen for a single person may not be suited for a family with children. Remember that owning a pet is a lifetime commitment.

3. What is your home like? Do you want your dog to be an inside dog, outside dog, or both?

Do you live in a small apartment, house with a fenced yard, etc.? Some dogs need lots of room and exercise (not just the big ones, some small breeds need lots of exercise). Will you be able to provide that space and exercise?

4. What pets do you already have? Are you planning on having other pets in the near future besides the dog?

Some dogs don't get along well with other animals (and vice versa). You should think very carefully before bringing a new dog into a household with other pets that she may not get along with.

5. What is your lifestyle like?

Are you very active and rarely home or fairly inactive and home most of the time or somewhere in between? Do you have activities that you want your dog to be a part of? Dogs are highly social animals and need companionship; however, some dogs may tolerate more isolation than others. If you are very active and rarely home perhaps you should consider another kind of pet.

6. What temperament do you want in your dog?

Do you want a very active dog or very inactive dog? Do you want one that is shy or very outgoing with strangers? What about a dog that demands a lot of attention? Is ease of obedience training important to you? A dog's temperament is very important to how well it will fit into your household. You should consider very carefully what temperament characteristics you want in your dog and then consult the books listed at the end of this handout to help pick a dog that has those characteristics.

7. What breed of dog do you want? Why?

Do you want a purebred dog or a mixed breed dog? Never pick a dog solely on its looks or its physical characteristics. It may not have the temperament or other characteristics you want. Consult books, breeders, your veterinarian, and friends who own a breed you are considering to help choose a breed. Consider a mixed breed dog from a shelter. They often have fewer physical and behavioral problems than do purebred dogs, but may be more of a gamble with an unknown history. If you buy a purebred dog, only buy from an established breeder with a good reputation.

8. What size dog do you want? Why?

Big dog, small dog, or in between? Different sized dogs have different abilities, characteristics, and needs.

9. What kind of coat characteristics and coat color do you want?

Some coats are more likely to shed than others, and some may require more care than others.

10. What sex dog do you want? Why?

Each sex has its own advantages and disadvantages, special needs and problems. Males are more likely to roam, urine mark, and fight with other dogs, for example. All dogs should be spayed or neutered unless you are planning to show the dog competitively or breed the dog. Spaying and neutering reduce the chances of certain behavioral and medical problems as well as reducing the pet overpopulation problem.

11. What age dog do you want? Why?

Puppies can be lots of fun but they can be a lot of work to housebreak, train, and socialize. Are you prepared to put in the work necessary to have a puppy?

12. Have you thought through the potential costs and problems associated with owning a dog?

Owning a dog can be a very rich and rewarding experience. However, along with the rewards come problems and costs. There will be a time commitment required; feeding, grooming, and healthcare costs; cleaning up after the dog; and some destruction of your property by the dog. Are you committed to dealing with these problems and costs? Remember that owning a dog is a lifetime commitment.

Some Books to Help You Choose a Dog

B. L. Hart and L. A. Hart, *The Perfect Puppy* (W.H. Freeman and Co., New York, 1988).

D. F. Tortora, *The Right Dog For You* (Simon and Schuster, New York, 1980).

Canine and Human Characteristics to Consider in Choosing a Dog

Dog Characteristics	Human Characteristics
Coat, shedding and grooming	Tolerance for shedding; willingness, time, and money to groom
Height, weight, bulkiness, and longevity	Desire for a big dog, environment for a big dog, money for a big dog, longevity expectations
Indoor and outdoor activity	Enjoyment of activity, restlessness
Vigor (gentle, rough vigorous)	Enjoyment of physical activity
Behavioral constancy (stick-to-itiveness)	Impulsiveness, responsibility
Dominance with familiar people and with unfamiliar people Territoriality	Dominance (leadership, assertiveness, initiative)
Emotional stability (high strung, nervous)	Emotionality, irritability
Sociability to familiar people, to unfamiliar people, to children Learning rate	Sociability, social desire, frequency of visitors and children; human acceptance or faultfinding

Dog Characteristics	Human Characteristics
Obedience	Desire for obedience
Problem solving ability	
Watch dog ability	Need for watch dog
Guard dog ability	Need for guard dog

From: B.L. Hart and L.A. Hart, 1988, *The Perfect Puppy;* D.F. Tortora, 1980, *The Right Dog for You.*

Puppy Class Outline

Week I

1. Handling/massage

People sit on floor with puppies (more than one/family can participate) and gently massage body, legs, paws. Progress to lifting lip, opening mouth briefly, squeezing paws, cradling in arms on back, putting finger in mouth, examining ears, etc. If puppy is fearful or aggressive, use tidbits to associate process with positive consequences.

2. Attention getting/calling puppy

Allow puppy to wander to end of six-foot leash. Bend down, use pup's name and call him in a happy excited, tone of voice. Do whatever it takes to get pup's attention—pat floor, clap hands, use a toy or tidbit. Praise pup when it comes. Practice with increasing distractions: let pup get involved in sniffing something, playing with another pup, etc., before calling it. Never call to punish or when coming will result in an aversive experience.

3. Sit

Hold a small tidbit (something soft which can be easily swallowed such as soft-moist dog food, a tiny piece of cheese, a hot dog, etc., *not* hard, crunchy treats) directly above pup's head. Pup should be looking up at the food. Move hand backward (not up), at same time using the command, "sit." As pup's head goes back, rear goes down. Give pup tidbit as soon as rear is on the floor. Try to get pup in position without touching him.

4. Discussion topics

Leash and collars—why no choke chains. Owners should be using the smallest leash possible; that is, width and size of snap.

Tell owners about development of social behavior, critical period (4–16 weeks).

Discuss goals/perspective of class. Can't expect same performance/attention from puppy as from older dog. Training, both in class and at home, will be positive reinforcement: distracting puppy from what you don't want it to do and encouraging and rewarding it to behave appropriately. Punishment is worst way to work with puppy problems.

Week II

1. Walking on leash/attention getting.

Goal is to have puppy walk with you on left side on a loose leash, paying attention to you. Proper heel position as in beginning class is not important. Continue using whatever stimuli are necessary to keep puppy's attention—slapping leg, toy, treats, praise, etc. Can use command such as "with me" or "by me" so as not confuse with more formal "heel" command later. If puppy leaves side, stop, call as in item 2 from first week, continue on. Do not jerk and pull. Tug on leash can be given to assist with attention getting.

2. Sound and texture experiences.

Expose puppy to several unfamiliar sounds and textures. These should be relatively easy ones; work up to more difficult/startling ones. Texture ideas include walking on newspaper, plastic, and Styrofoam shipping "peanuts." Sounds include party noisemaker, class applauding, cheering, and popping paper bag.

3. Continue handling experiences.

Handling should progress to more restraint, examination of feet, mouth, ears in addition to gentle massage and touching. Discuss grooming while doing. Puppy should also be handled by at least one person it does not know. This handling should be very gentle, more like first week.

4. Continue with "sit."

If puppy is performing well at home, begin to "wean off" treats gradually. Sometimes use treat, sometimes not. Add a brief "stay" to sit—not like in beginning class. Owner will probably already be in front of puppy. Have owner use hand signal along with verbal command; pup should stay 5 to 10 seconds before release. Owner should not try to back away from pup this week. Teach importance of specific release word.

5. Discussion topics.

"Puppy-proofing" house, destructive behavior, crate training, housetraining.

Week III

1. Continue with walking on leash, attention. Add sit at halt.

Work on changing directions. Precise heeling is not important. Pup should be paying attention, staying on loose leash close to owner so can follow change of direction. Begin having pup sit when stopped. "Straight sit" in heel position not important.

2. Continue with recall.

During walking on leash practice, instructors can take one pup at a time, hold pup's leash while owner walks 8–10 feet away and calls pup, who must pass by a few other puppies to get to owner. Owner should bend down, call excitedly, use food, toy, whatever. Should not be a formal recall.

3. Teach "down."

Use tidbit technique. Begin by having pup sit. Have tidbit, hold in front of pup's nose, move hand straight down to floor, then forward. This encourages pup to do the same. Some pup's rear ends will come up (especially short legged breeds). Owner can use other hand to hold rear down. As soon as pup is down, it gets treat. For difficult pups, use shaping procedure and reward for part of movement. With each successive attempt, must move more toward down. Discuss commands "down" and "off."

4. Sound/texture experiences.

Add chicken wire, walk through pan of shallow warm water. Sounds: drop a book, hit metal pan with spoon, fan. For all of these experiences, sounds should start quietly and then increase in volume. If pup startles, move it farther away from sound. Elicit nonfearful behavior with treats, toys, praise.

5. Socialization experiences.

Puppies should be introduced to other people. Either "pass the puppy" around a circle or switch puppies and do easy work on leash walking, coming, sitting. Should all be very positive and gentle. Also allow puppies to interact with each other more.

6. Discussion topics.

Chewing, separation anxiety, mouthing/nipping, jumping up—have pup sit for attention instead. Discuss no punishment after the fact, misinterpretation of "guilty looks."

Week IV

1. Work on "stay."

Add "stay" to "down," similar to "sit." Owner should stay with pup, use hand signal, have pup hold position for 5–15 seconds. Owner can begin backing away a few steps on sit-stay. Work on getting pup to lie down without intermediate sit position.

2. Round robin recalls.

Class sits on floor. Work with two to four puppies at a time. Exchange puppies, handle, massage, then owner calls back across circle.

3. Walking on leash.

Work on stairs, passing between others, up to wall, in narrow area by couch, over an obstacle. Continue attention getting, sit at halt.

4. Sound/texture experiences.

Pass through a cardboard box/tunnel, balloons, sirens, gunshot/firecrackers (from sound effects album).

5. Work with sit-stand-sit-down sequence with tidbit.

From Ian Dunbar's tape. Use food, moving hand to have pup change positions from sit to stand (move hand forward) to sit to down.

6. Exposure to new people.

Several people can be assigned to come in uniform (if used in their jobs); make sure pups meet children. Instructors or others can bring large hats, sunglasses, wigs, beards.

6. Discussion topics

Grooming, spay/neuter. Cover myths and also what behaviors neutering does affect (urine marking, roaming, *some* forms of aggression, mounting).

Week V

1. Retrieving.

Work with short distances, in a corner or against a wall, to encourage pup to bring toy back. Work on getting pup to drop toy, in exchange for a food reward if necessary. Also discuss tug-of-war, wrestling games, limiting number of toys.

2. Continue with "stay."

Owner can also back away from pup on down-stay. Add a brief, 5–10 second stay to stand. Work sit-stand-sit-down sequence.

3. Drop leash "heelinq."

Owners should continue walking on leash as before. When pup is paying attention and doing well, drop leash. Not having leash in hand often forces owners to work harder to keep pup's attention rather than relying on leash. If pup wanders away, owner should bend down, call pup and start again.

4. "Not paid for" exercise.

Pup learns not to take treat until owner says, "Okay."

5. Discussion topics

Expectations—although pup may now be looking like an adult in physical appearance, is not adult behaviorally. Still has short attention span, is curious, and is not to be trusted. Discuss appearance of some behavior problems at time of sexual maturity (e.g., about two years, dominance aggression).

If time, can teach one or two easy tricks such as shake hands, jump over, or roll over. (lot depends on size and maturity of pup).

Week VI

Puppy party

Encourage owners to come in costume for additional socialization for puppies. Demonstrate beginning obedience exercises, tricks. Encourage owners to continue with beginning class.

Allow puppies to interact with each other and other people. Distribute certificates, ribbons. Could have prize for quickest sit, longest stay, best trick, or whatever.

Crate Training Your Dog

How quickly a dog will adapt to a crate will depend on her age, temperament, and previous experiences. Crate training may only take a few days or as long as several weeks. The crate should always be associated with something pleasant for the dog. Training should take place in a series of small steps—don't try to do too much too fast.

Step 1: Introducing Your Dog to the Crate

Put the crate in an area of the house where the family spends a lot of time, such as the den or kitchen. Put a soft sleeping blanket or towel in the crate. Bring your dog over to the crate and talk to him in an excited, happy tone of voice. Make sure the door to the crate is securely fastened opened so it won't accidentally hit your dog and frighten him.

Drop some small tidbits of food around the crate, just inside the door, and then gradually all the way inside the crate to encourage your dog to enter. If he doesn't go all the way in at first to get the food, that's okay. *Do not* force him to enter. Repeat this experience until your dog will calmly walk into the crate to get the food. If your dog isn't interested in food, try tossing a favorite toy in the crate instead. This process may take just a few minutes or as long as several days.

Step 2: Feeding Your Dog in the Crate

After your dog has been introduced to the crate as in Step 1, you can begin feeding him his regular meals near or in the crate for awhile. This will create pleasant associations with the crate and decrease any fear he has of the crate. If your dog is readily entering the crate when you begin Step 2, you can place the food dish all the way at the back of the crate. However, if your dog is still reluctant to enter the crate, then place the dish right in front of the open door or as far inside as he will readily go without becoming fearful or anxious. Each time you feed him, place the dish a little more toward the back of the crate.

Once your dog is comfortably eating his food while standing in the crate, you can close the door while he's eating. At first, open the door as soon as he finishes his meal, let him out, and praise him. With each succeeding feeding, leave the door closed a few minutes longer, until he is staying in the crate without protesting for 10 minutes or so after eating. If he begins to whine to be let out, you may have increased the duration of crating too quickly. Next time, try leaving him for a shorter time period. Be sure to release him from the crate when he is not whining or barking. If he is let out while he's making noise, noisy behavior is reinforced and he'll be more likely to make noise the next time.

Step 3: Conditioning Your Dog to Stay in the Crate for Longer Time Periods

After your dog is eating his regular meals in the crate with no sign of fear or anxiety, you can begin to confine him there for short time periods while you are home. Begin by calling him over to the crate in return for a food reward. Give him a command to enter, such as "kennel up." You can encourage him to enter by pointing to the inside of the crate with a tidbit in your hand. After your dog enters the crate, reward him with the tidbit and close the door. Sit quietly near the crate for 5–10 minutes and then go out of sight into another room for a few minutes. When you return, sit quietly again for a short time, and then release your dog. Repeat this procedure several times a day. With each repetition, gradually increase the length of time the dog is crated and the length of time you are out of sight. Once your dog will quietly remain in the crate for about 30 minutes with you out of sight the majority of the time, you can begin leaving him crated when you are gone for short time periods, and/or letting him sleep there at night. It may take several days or several weeks to get to this point.

Step 4: Crating—Alone or at Night
Part A—Crating When Left Alone

After your dog is spending about 30 minutes in the crate without becoming anxious or afraid while you are home, you can begin leaving him crated for short time periods when you leave the house. Put him in the crate with your regular "kennel up" (or similar) command. You will want to vary at what point you put your dog in the crate during your "getting ready to leave" routine. Although he should not be crated for a long time before you leave, you can crate him anywhere from 5 to 20 minutes prior to leaving. Do not make departures or arrivals emotional and prolonged, but matter-of-fact instead. Praise your dog briefly and give him a tidbit for entering the crate and then leave quietly. When you arrive home do not inadvertently reward your dog for excited behavior by responding to him in an excited, enthusiastic way. Keep arrivals very low key and reserve playful, excited greeting behavior for after he has been let outside and has calmed down somewhat. Continue to crate your dog for short time periods from time to time when you are home so that he does not begin to associate crating with being left alone.

Step 4
Part B—Crating at Night

Follow the same procedure you have been using to encourage your dog to enter his crate willingly. Initially, it may be a good idea (especially if you have a young puppy) to locate the crate in your bedroom or nearby in a hallway. Puppies often need to go outside to eliminate at night, and you'll want to be able to hear your puppy when he whines to be let outside. Older dogs too should initially be kept nearby so that crating does not become associated with social isolation. Once your dog is sleeping comfortably through the night with his crate near you, you can begin to gradually move it to the location you prefer.

If Your Dog Whines or Cries

If your dog whines or cries while in the crate at night, it may be difficult to decide whether he is whining just because he wants out of the crate, of whether he needs to be let outside to eliminate. Whining is more likely to be caused by social isolation if the crate is located in another room. First, try moving the crate to your bedroom or close by.

If you followed the training procedures, your dog should not have been reinforced for whining by being released from his crate. Initially you can ignore the whining. Your dog may stop if he is just testing you. Yelling at him or pounding on the crate may only increase his vocalizations and may make him fearful. If the whining continues after you have ignored it for several minutes, you can repeat the phrase your dog has associated with going outside to eliminate. If he responds and becomes excited, take him outside. This should be a trip with a purpose, not play time. If you are convinced your dog does not need to eliminate, the best response is to ignore the whining until it stops. Most attempts at punishing the behavior actually end up inadvertently reinforcing the noise because the dog is getting attention from you. When you ignore the whining, expect it to get worse before it gets better. You cannot give in, otherwise you will teach your dog that he must whine louder and longer to get what he wants. If you have progressed very gradually through the training steps and have not attempted to hurry the process, you will be less likely to encounter this problem. If additional problems arise, contact your veterinarian for more information or for a referral to a behavior specialist. Animal Behavior Associates, Inc., will be happy to consult with you and help you with your pet.

Housetraining Procedures for Puppies and Adult Dogs

One of the reasons that we can keep dogs and cats as house pets is because their elimination behavior patterns allow them to be trained to go to the bathroom in locations which are acceptable to us. However, puppies cannot be expected to control their bladder and bowels for long time periods until five to six months of age. Some puppies are not fully housetrained until they are eight or nine months or even a year old. Because dogs are denning animals, like wolves, they tend not to soil the area they consider to be their den. You cannot assume that your new adult dog or puppy will realize at first that your entire house is now his den. You must teach him that. This handout provides information about basic housetraining procedures.

Housetraining Puppies

1. Establish a routine.

Housetraining a puppy requires time and commitment from you. The more consistent you are, the quicker your puppy will learn acceptable behavior. Like babies, puppies do best on a regular schedule. If possible, put your puppy on a regular feeding schedule. Check with your veterinarian, but depending on its age, puppies usually need to be fed three or four times a day. Feeding your puppy at consistent times will make it more likely that she will need to go to the bathroom at consistent time periods as well. This will make housetraining much easier.

2. Reward good behavior.

Take your puppy outside frequently, at least every two hours. Your puppy should also be taken outside when she wakes up from a nap, after playing, and after eating. Establish two command phrases, one which asks "Do you need to go outside?" and another which says "Go do your business!" once outside. Use whatever words you choose, but *be consistent—always use the exact same phrase.* Go outside with your puppy. Repeat your command phrase, and when she urinates or defecates, praise your puppy quietly but enthusiastically. Also give your pup a tidbit as a reward for eliminating outside. Most pet owners forget to reward puppies for doing the right thing. The importance of rewarding good behavior (rather than punishing unacceptable behavior) cannot be overemphasized.

3. Supervise your puppy.

A new puppy must be supervised constantly. Puppies who are allowed to wander off into rooms by themselves or who are left alone, free in the house, will most likely get into trouble. Always be sure you know where your puppy is. Encourage her to stay in the same room with you or another family member. You can "tether" her to you on a six-foot leash or use baby gates to keep her in the room where you are. Close doors to unoccupied rooms. When a puppy must be left alone for relatively long time periods, she should be confined in a small area or a crate. This area, or crate, must be large enough to provide a sleeping and playing area, as well as an area where the puppy can eliminate. Papers can be placed in that part of the confinement area designated as okay for the puppy to eliminate in. Because young puppies cannot always control their bladder and bowels for long time periods, it is not fair to confine a puppy for an entire work day with no place to relieve itself. A puppy can be crated at night (preferably in the same room with a family member) if you are willing to get up and go outside with her when necessary. A handout about crate training is also available from us.

4. Never punish after the fact.

Virtually every puppy will have an accident in the house. Expect this; it is part of owning a puppy. If—*and only if*—you catch your puppy in the act of soiling, do something that startles her, which she will perceive as coming from the environment, not from you. Make a loud noise (slap your palm against the wall, drop something) or toss a pillow toward your puppy. ***Do not rub your puppy's nose in the mess or hit her.*** This will teach your puppy to be afraid of you and afraid to eliminate in your presence—and you do want her to go to the bathroom in the yard when you are there. If you find a soiled area but do not catch your puppy soiling, do nothing but clean it up. Animals do not understand punishment after the fact, even if it is only seconds. Punishment after the fact without a doubt will do more harm than good. Punishment should punish the behavior, not the animal. This cannot happen unless the puppy is caught in the act.

5. Use enzymatic cleaners.

The best cleaning agents to use for soiled areas are the enzymatic type cleaners available at many pet stores. The enzymes break up the organic material which produces the odor. Do not clean with ammonia, as this smells similar to urine. Vinegar diluted with water can also help neutralize odor. If your puppy has picked a favorite spot to soil, not only should it be thoroughly cleaned, but it can be made less appealing by changing the texture. You can do this by covering it with plastic, or tape which is sticky on both sides. However, you must also make sure that you are following all the rest of the basic housetraining procedures, especially *rewarding your puppy for going outside.*

6. Provide more freedom gradually.

As your puppy matures and begins to show you that it understands going outside to eliminate is what you expect, you can gradually increase her freedom. If you wish, you can leave her free in the house for short time periods, while you run to the store, for example. Don't expect her to make the transition from being confined to being left completely free in the house in a single step.

When Adult Dogs Need Retraining

Dogs obtained from previous owners or animal shelters may have been housetrained in their previous homes. However, this does not guarantee that this will be the case in their new homes. Shelter dogs have no choice but to eliminate in their runs or cages, which may weaken good housetrained habits. The routine and physical environment in a new household will be different from the previous one, so a dog may not know for a while how to get outside or how to let his new owners know what he wants. When first in a new environment, a dog may not yet realize that this is now his den. Even spayed and neutered animals may also want to urine-mark their new territory for awhile. Scents and odors from previous pets can also stimulate urine marking.

For the first few days and weeks, you should assume that your new dog is *not* housetrained. Treat her just as you would a puppy: establish a regular schedule, take her outside frequently, reward her for eliminating outside, and supervise her activity while inside. Progress should be much faster than with a puppy because you are refreshing and reinforcing already established habits, rather than teaching totally new behaviors.

Common Causes of House Soiling Problems

If you have consistently followed basic housetraining procedures and your dog continues to eliminate in the house, then the cause of the behavior must be determined before it can be changed. There are other reasons why dogs house soil other than a lack of housetraining. Some examples of causes of house soiling are

- *Medical problems.* House soiling can often be caused by physical problems such as a urinary tract infection or an irritated bowel. Check with your veterinarian to rule out any possibility of disease or illness.
- *Territorial urine marking.* Dogs will deposit urine, usually in small amounts, to scent-mark territory. Both male and female dogs may do this. This most often occurs when the dog believes its territory has been invaded.
- *Separation anxiety.* It is not uncommon for dogs to become anxious when left alone and house soil as a result. If the soiling is occurring only, and consistently, when your dog is left alone, separation anxiety may be the cause.
- *Fears or phobias.* When animals become frightened, they often lose control of their bladders and/or bowels. If your dog is afraid of loud noises, thunderstorms, or other things, it may house soil when exposed to these environmental events.
- *Submissive/excitement urination.* Some dogs, especially young ones, temporarily lose control of their bladders when they become excited or threatened. This usually occurs during greetings, intense play, or when they are about to be punished (another good reason for not punishing after the fact or using physical types of punishment).

The techniques necessary to correct a house soiling problem depend on the cause. If your veterinarian has determined your dog does not have a medical problem, the certified applied animal behaviorists at Animal Behavior Associates, Inc., will be happy to consult with you and help you work with your dog.

Preventing Destructive Behavior by Puppies

The first thing you should know is that chewing and digging by puppies are perfectly natural, normal behaviors. It is unlikely that anything you do will stop these behaviors completely. What we will try to do is give you some things to do to lessen the damage. You should accept the fact that if you own a dog you will experience property damage and lose something of value. The basic strategies in preventing puppy damage are to (1) prevent access to things that you don't want damaged or make those things give the animal an unpleasant experience when she tries to damage them and (2) to provide acceptable things to chew and places to dig.

Puppy Chewing

Puppies are very oral beings. One of the main ways they explore their world is to put things in their mouths and chew on them. Teething occurs in puppies up to six to eight months of age. This can make chewing problems even worse in young animals.

- Puppy proof your house. This means keeping things that can be destroyed out of reach of the animal. Keep clothes, children's toys, and other small objects off the floor. Keep closets, drawers, and toy boxes closed any time the puppy is out. Remove objects from lower shelves, end tables, or any other surface the puppy can reach.
- Keep a close watch on your puppy. Never let your puppy run loose in the house without supervision. If there are times you cannot watch the puppy, put her in a secure area like a kitchen with baby gates at the doors to prevent escapes, in a dog exercise pen, or in a crate or dog kennel. (If you use a crate or kennel be sure that the dog has been properly crate trained. To do otherwise may create other problems.) You could also leash the dog to your belt to keep her out of mischief.
- For objects that may be chewed that you cannot prevent your puppy from gaining access to, try to make them aversive by coating the surfaces with Bitter Apple, a hot sauce, or Listerine mouthwash (be sure the surface is color fast and that the material will not damage the surface). For other things that cannot be treated in this way, make the areas around the objects unpleasant by putting down plastic rug runner (pointy side up), motion detectors such as The Scraminal, or vibration sensors such as The Tattle Tale. Be consistent in discouraging chewing of inappropriate objects. *Never* encourage it.
- If you catch your puppy chewing some inappropriate object, tell her "no," take it away from her, and give her an appropriate chew object. *Never* punish your puppy for chewing things after the fact. Punishment is neither effective nor appropriate if you don't catch the animal in the act.
- Provide plenty of acceptable chew toys such as Nylabones, Kong Toys, cattle hooves, sterilized large beef bones, or rawhide chewies (check with your veterinarian about what are safe, acceptable chew toys). You may have to experiment with different objects to find ones that your puppy likes. Praise and reward your puppy for chewing appropriate things.
- *Never* give your puppy old clothes, shoes, or children's toys as chew toys. The puppy may not learn the difference between them and your good clothes, shoes, etc.
- If these things don't help, or if the destructiveness gets worse, consult a professional for help.

Puppy Digging

- Puppy proof your yard, garden and flower beds, and any indoor area that may be scratched such as doors, carpets and rugs. Put up fences or other barriers to keep her out of unwanted areas.

• Booby trap other areas that the puppy cannot be kept out of. Fill in holes and stretch hardware cloth over the area to make it unpleasant to dig. Inside, put out plastic carpet runner, Scat Mat, or other devices to make scratched areas unpleasant to scratch.

• For a puppy that is strongly motivated to dig, set aside a part of your yard for her to dig in, and reward digging in that area.

• Seek professional help if the digging continues or gets worse.

When Puppies and Kittens Eat Things They Shouldn't

Definitions

Puppies and kittens will sometimes eat or merely suckle on clothing or other objects which may result in a variety of problems for both owners and animals. Not only can the owner's possessions be destroyed, but clothing and other objects can produce life-threatening blockages in the animal's intestines. Another form of this behavior, stool eating, while not necessarily dangerous to the animal is often unacceptable to the owner. Stool-eating is called *coprophagy,* and eating nonfood items is referred to as *pica.*

Causes

The causes of pica and coprophagy are not known. It has been suggested that coprophagy is carried over from the normal parental behavior of ingesting the waste of young offspring. However, puppies and kittens have obviously never had litters so this explanation seems not to apply to them. Some experts believe coprophagy occurs more often in animals who may be frequently confined to small areas and receive limited attention from their owners. Coprophagy may be seen more often in dogs who tend to be highly motivated by food. It is possible that a dog may learn this behavior from another dog. Coprophagy is fairly common in dogs and puppies but is rarely seen in cats, for reasons unknown. Both pica and coprophagy may be attempts to obtain a necessary nutrient lacking in the diet, although no nutritional studies have ever substantiated this idea. These behaviors may also be frustration or anxiety related and occur when the animal is "bored," anxious, or afraid. It is possible the behaviors begin as play, as the animal investigates and chews on the objects, and subsequently, for unknown reasons, begins to eat or ingest them. Suckling of objects seems to occur more frequently in cats than in dogs. Weaning a kitten too soon may contribute to or cause this problem.

Coprophagy

Stopping Coprophagy

Because the causes of the problem are not well understood, no treatments that are consistently successful are available. A commercial product, 4-BID, available from veterinarians, when put on a dog's food supposedly produces a stool with an unpleasant taste. It has been said the same result can be achieved by putting

MSG (monosodiumglutamate, a food additive) or meat tenderizer on the food. Based on owners' reports, both of these products appear to work in some cases, but are often ineffective. Before using either of these products, check with your veterinarian. The stools can also be given an aversive taste by sprinkling them directly with either cayenne pepper or a commercial product called Bitter Apple. For this method to be effective, every stool the animal has access to for a length of time must be treated in order for him to learn that eating stools results in unpleasant consequences. It is obviously difficult for most owners to watch their dogs each and every time they defecate. In addition, it may be possible for some dogs to discriminate by odor which stools have been treated and which have not. Interactive punishment (punishment which comes from the owner) is usually not effective because (1) attempts at punishment, such as a verbal scolding, may be interpreted by the dog as attention and/or (2) many dogs learn not to show the behavior when their owners are present, but will do so when owners are absent. The simplest solution may simply be to clean the yard daily in order to minimize the dog's opportunity for coprophagy. Puppies may outgrow the behavior.

Any type of environmental booby trap to stop a puppy from eating cat feces from the litter box must be attempted with caution. Anything which frightens a puppy away from a litter box is also likely to frighten the cat away as well. It is much better to install a baby gate in front of the litter box area as a cat will have no trouble jumping over it while most puppies will not make the attempt. Alternatively, the box can be placed in a closet or room where the door can be wedged open from both sides (so the cat cannot be trapped in or out) a small enough distance to allow the cat access but not the puppy.

Health Risks

In Colorado's dry climate, parasites are not nearly the problem as in other parts of the country. A dog who is parasite free and is eating only his own stools cannot be infected with parasites by doing so. If a dog is eating the stools of another dog who has parasites, it may be possible, although still unlikely, for the dog to become infected. Some parasites, such as giardia, cause diarrhea, and most coprophagic dogs ingest only formed stools. In addition, there is a delay period before the parasites in the stools can infect another animal. Finally, most parasites require intermediate hosts (they must pass through the body of another species such as a flea) before they can infect another dog or cat. Thus, dogs are much more likely to become infected with parasites through fleas and killing and/or eating birds and rodents than by coprophagy. Most parasites are also species specific, meaning that dogs cannot be infected by eating cat stools. Although some owners may think it unpleasant, health risks to humans from being licked in the face by a coprophagic dog are minimal. For more information, contact your veterinarian.

Pica

Pica can be a more serious problem that coprophagy because items such as rubber bands and string can severely damage or block an animal's intestines. In some instances, the items must be surgically removed. The chances of resolving this type of problem successfully will probably be greater if the reason for the behavior can be determined. Unfortunately, this will often not be possible as the behavior is poorly understood. Making the objects the animal is eating taste unpleasant with some of the substances mentioned previously may be helpful. Owners may need to prevent the animal's access to the items and/or be very vigilant about putting socks and other such items out of reach. If the animal is very food oriented, it may be possible to change to a low-calorie or high-fiber diet to allow him to eat more food more often, which may decrease the behavior. Check with your veterinarian before changing diets.

Pica can be an attention-getting behavior, play behavior, or a frustration or anxiety-relieving behavior. If anxiety or frustration are involved, the reason for these reactions must be identified and the behavior changed using behavior modification techniques. For attention-getting behaviors, the animal can be startled with a loud noise or a spray of water when she is caught ingesting the items, and should receive attention and social interaction from the owner when the items are left alone. Cats commonly play with string, rubber bands, and tinsel and ultimately ingest them. Owners need to keep these items out of reach and provide a selection of appropriate toys.

Because pica can potentially be a life-threatening behavior problem, it may be advisable to consult *both* your veterinarian and a behavior professional for help.

Suckling Behavior

Young kittens may suckle on the owner's hair, fingers, toys, clothing or other objects such as blankets and bedding. Most often, kittens showing such behavior may have been weaned too young. The items can either be made to taste unpleasant using products previously mentioned and/or the kitten can be distracted with a toy when caught suckling. An acceptable item for suckling, such as a doll's baby bottle, may be provided until the kitten matures.

There are various reports in the behavior literature of Siamese and Siamese mixed-breed cats showing a tendency to suckle on and sometimes ingest woolen objects. This problem is not exclusive to this breed however, as it occurs in other breeds as well. The reason for this behavior is unknown. It has been suggested that the cat may be attracted to the odor of lanolin in the wool, but this idea has not been proven or even widely accepted by cat behavior experts. Not allowing the cat to have access to wool items, treating them with an unpleasant tasting substance as mentioned above, or startling the cat with a loud noise or water sprayer when caught may all be helpful.

Punishment Is Counterproductive

Punishment after the fact for any of these behaviors is *never* helpful. This approach will *not* resolve the problem and is likely to produce either fearful or aggressive responses from the animal. If your puppy or kitten is displaying pica or coprophagy, ask your veterinarian for more information or for a referral to a behavior specialist. The certified applied animal behaviorists at Animal Behavior Associates, Inc., will be happy to consult with you and help you work with your pet.

Preventing Aggressive Behavior by Puppies

Aggression by dogs directed at people is the most serious problem faced by owners. Aggressive dogs can cause serious injury or even death. There is nothing that an owner can do that will absolutely guarantee that a puppy will never become aggressive. This is because our knowledge about the causes of aggression is incomplete. However, there are some things that you can do as an owner that will lessen the likelihood that your puppy will become aggressive. Some of these are designed to prevent puppy aggression, while others are designed to prevent aggression as your dog grows up.

Genetics and Breeding

Genetics and breeding can influence aggression and other problem behaviors.

- If you buy a puppy, purchase it from an established breeder with a good reputation. Always ask the breeder about the parents and brothers and sisters of the puppy. Never buy a puppy that has been bred to be aggressive or whose parents or siblings have been aggressive or fearful of people. Be sure that the puppy has had plenty of contact with people and other dogs. Avoid buying puppies that seem overly excitable or overly fearful.
- If you get a dog from a shelter or pet store where you cannot ask about the parents or siblings, don't pick a dog that is overly excitable or overly fearful. Avoid getting a dog that has been living by itself with little contact with other dogs or people.

Out of Control Play

Out of control play is one of the most common causes of injury by puppies. Puppies should always be encouraged to play gently with people.

- *Never* encourage a puppy to play roughly and to bite or mouth clothing or skin. This only rewards unacceptable behavior. Children should be taught acceptable ways to play with puppies and supervised to be sure that they are not encouraging bad behavior.
- If the puppy tries to bite, nip, or play roughly, (1) try to direct her play onto a ball, chew toy, or other appropriate toy, (2) put the puppy on a time-out for a few minutes away from people, or (3) use remote punishment to discourage rough play. Remote punishment means telling the puppy "no" at the same time you squirt her with water or make a loud startling sound like shaking a can full of pennies. The punishment should always occur during the rough play, never after. If you cannot catch her in the act, don't punish her. *Never* hit, slap, kick, or use other physical punishment with a puppy. It is unnecessary and may make the problem worse.
- Always try to make touching, petting, and grooming the puppy a calm, relaxed, and nonplayful situation. Encouraging play in these situations will only make it more difficult for the puppy to learn the difference between play and nonplay situations.

Fear and Pain

Fear and pain are the other major causes of puppies injuring people.

- *Never* hit, slap, kick, or hurt a puppy. It is cruel and may cause the puppy to bite or become fearful of you.
- Young children should never be left alone with puppies or allowed to hurt or scare them.
- Never scare puppies with loud noises, sudden movements, or other frightening events.
- If your puppy is frightened of sounds, things (like vacuum cleaners), or people, get professional help.

Dominance Aggression

Dominance aggression is one of the most common causes of aggression in adult dogs. It occurs when the dog tries to dominate one or more members of the household.

- Neutering male dogs and spaying female dogs may reduce the likelihood of dominance aggression developing.
- Puppies should be taught to tolerate handling, being restrained, petted, groomed, and moved around as well as having food, toys, and chew bones taken from them. Rewards, *not force,* should be used to get the puppy to comply so that she has a good attitude about doing these things. These activities should be done regularly as a normal part of play, feeding, grooming, etc.
- It is *not* necessary to "scruff shake," roll a puppy over and pin it to the ground, or use other dog dominance gestures to reinforce your dominance over the puppy.
- Simple rules should be developed by the family as to what the puppy can and can't do around the house (such as sleeping on the bed, getting on the furniture, getting food scraps from the table, etc.). These rules should be enforced consistently by all family members.
- Punishment for misbehavior of any sort should be done only when other things have been tried and have failed. Punishment should only be of the remote kind (a loud noise, water squirted on the puppy, or a small pillow thrown in the general direction of the puppy, *don't* hit the puppy with the pillow).

Possessive Aggression

Possessive aggression occurs when a dog thinks that a person is trying to take something away from her that she values such as food, a toy, or a chew bone.

- Puppies should be taught to tolerate having food, toys, and chew bones taken from them. Rewards, *not force,* should be used to get the puppy to comply so that she has a good attitude about doing these things. These activities should be done regularly as a normal part of play, feeding, grooming, etc.
- Never punish a puppy for not giving up these objects. Trade the puppy a food treat or other toy for things it will not readily give up.

Territorial and Protective Aggression

Territorial and protective aggression occurs when a dog tries to drive away unfamiliar people or dogs from her territory or from people or dogs she is attached to.

- Puppies should be socialized with other dogs and unfamiliar people. This means gradual, nonthreatening exposure associated with rewards (food, play, petting) while your dog is nonaggressive, nonfearful, relaxed, and comfortable. A good puppy class can help with this and help prevent many other problems.
- Puppies should be taught to be calm and quiet when people or dogs pass by your property (including your car), come on your property, or come into your house. Use food or other rewards to get your dog to sit or lie down quietly.
- Puppies should be taught to be calm and quiet when people or dogs approach you or other family members while on walks or otherwise away from your home.
- Physical punishment should not be used to stop puppies that are barking, threatening, or out of control around unfamiliar people or dogs.

Predatory Behavior

Predatory behavior occurs when dogs attempt to hunt and kill small animals like cats, squirrels, or birds.

- Puppies should *never* be encouraged to hunt small animals or birds or to excitedly chase any animal or person.
- Puppies caught in the act of stalking, chasing, or lunging at people or other animals should be discouraged by loudly approaching them, making a loud sound, or squirting them with water.
- Puppies should never be punished after the fact for stalking, chasing, or lunging or for carrying or consuming prey.
- Restrict the puppy's access to small animals and birds to prevent predation.

Get Professional Help

If an aggression problem develops, get professional help immediately, do not wait. It is very likely that the longer you wait, the worse the problem will become.

If you find yourself punishing your dog more than just occasionally, seek professional help to deal with the problem.

Introducing Your New Puppy to Your Other Dogs

Dogs are social animals. This means they normally live together in groups that are highly structured. A dominance hierarchy or "pecking order" is established among dogs living in the same household. This order is determined by the outcomes of interactions between the dogs. Owners cannot choose which dog they want to be dominant. When a new dog is brought into the family, the hierarchy is upset and becomes unstable as the newcomer finds her own place in the social order.

Puppies and the Dominance Hierarchy

Puppies almost without exception will be the most subordinate members of the hierarchy. Within the litter, puppies will establish some degree of dominance hierarchy among themselves, but all will be submissive to adults. When you bring a new puppy into the house, expect the resident adult dog to establish herself as the dominant animal. Dominant dogs expect to receive certain benefits due to their social position. These can include being fed first, passing through doors first, being able to push other dogs out of the way in order to be petted, and controlling toys and preferred sleeping areas. These behaviors relate to social dominance, not to "jealousy" between the dogs, which is an anthropomorphic interpretation. Owners need to support the resident dog's position by allowing her to be first and not favoring the puppy. A dominant adult dog should also be allowed to set limits with the puppy by growling or snarling. Well socialized adult dogs with good temperaments will use these threatening behaviors to set limits with the puppy without harming her. These *ritualized* behaviors are the means dogs use to establish and maintain the social structure without injury to themselves or other members of the group. Preventing the adult dog from demonstrating her position using just threats can push her to show her dominance with more aggressive behaviors such as biting.

Keep the Routine

Keep the resident dog's routine the same as much as possible by not changing her feeding, exercise, play, and sleeping times and locations. You can also give both the adult and the puppy some time alone with you. It's not uncommon for a puppy to have a difficult time playing with toys because the adult dog takes his toys away. Either different family members can play with the animals in separate rooms at times, or the adult can be confined with a special chew toy while the puppy has some play time. Be careful not to isolate the adult in such a way that she perceives the puppy is receiving special attention and she is not. This could undermine the dominance hierarchy and contribute to a problem. Be sure to give an adult dog some quiet time away from the pestering play of a young puppy.

Initial Introduction

If you have chosen a puppy several days before he will actually come home, you can introduce your resident dog to the puppy's scent. Bring the puppy's sleeping blankets home from the breeder, or even just wipe a towel over the puppy you have chosen from the animal shelter. Put the towel under your dog's food bowl, in her bed, or in your lap when you hold her. In this way, the puppy's scent becomes associated with "good things" for the adult.

This idea—that the adult should expect "good things" to happen whenever the puppy is around—should be carried over to the rest of the introduction process. Let the resident dog sniff the puppy, which is normal canine greeting behavior. As she does so, talk to her in a happy, friendly tone of voice, "Look at your new friend! What a good dog you are!" Don't use a threatening tone of voice "Fidoooo—Be good." If you see the puppy becoming frightened or the adult getting too threatening, interrupt the interaction by getting the adult interested in doing something else. Call her over to you for a tidbit or toss her favorite ball. After both animals have calmed down, try the introduction again with more distance between the two dogs.

You may need to feed the dogs separately at first so the adult doesn't steal the puppy's food. The adult dog can also be encouraged to leave the puppy's food alone by giving her something else to do while the puppy is eating.

Introducing the Puppy to Several Resident Dogs

A group of dogs may have a tendency to "gang up" on a newcomer. In addition, *redirected* aggression can occur. If one of the adults is provoked by a more dominant one, he can attack a third, more subordinate animal, which may be the puppy. A puppy is a likely candidate for both kinds of attack. To be safe, if there is more than one resident dog, it's probably a good idea to introduce them to the puppy one at a time.

As the Puppy Matures

Aggressive fighting problems are unlikely to occur when a young puppy is first introduced because puppies are generally subordinate and not viewed by adults as threats. However, as the puppy matures and grows, she may attempt to challenge one or more of the adult dogs for a higher position in the social hierarchy. These "canine rivalry" problems need to be dealt with using appropriate behavioral techniques. Punishing either dog is likely to make the problem worse. If the introduction of your puppy does not go well or if conflicts between the dogs arise later on, consult your veterinarian for more information or for a referral to a behavior professional. The certified applied animal behaviorists at Animal Behavior Associates Inc., will be happy to consult with you and help you work with your dogs.

Introducing Your New Puppy to Your Cat

Dogs and cats who were not exposed to each other's species when they were young will require some extra time to become accustomed to each other. A puppy will likely want to play with an adult cat, or may even be afraid of her. An adult cat may react fearfully and defensively when confronted with a young, silly puppy, or she may decide to "take him on" if he gets too out of control. It is less likely for a puppy than an adult dog to respond aggressively to a cat, with the intent to harm her. Dogs and cats will react to each other differently because they differ in their communication signals and social behaviors. They will need to be introduced to each other slowly and gradually so that neither is harmed or frightened and aggressive reactions don't become a habit.

Introducing a Puppy to a Resident Cat

Step 1

Any puppy in a new home needs lots of supervision. Managing normal puppy behaviors such as housetraining and chewing require that the puppy not be allowed to explore the house unsupervised. Puppies, like toddlers, easily get into trouble on their own! Thus, when you first bring the puppy home, you'll want to choose an area where you can confine him when you can't be watching him. A kitchen or laundry room blocked off with a baby gate or other barrier works well. You can also use an exercise pen, a playpen, or a crate. Ask your veterinarian for a handout on crating and crate training to prevent overuse of the crate. Provide a bed, water, toys, food (if feeding free-choice), and papers for elimination if you are paper training the puppy.

Step 2

Unless the puppy is extremely rambunctious or the cat quite timid and frightened, you can probably let the cat decide on her own how close she wants to approach the puppy when he is confined in his area. If either animal becomes aggressive or frightened (a few hisses and barks are okay), you can manage the introduction by having one person sit with the puppy and offer him some small tidbits of food. Another person can sit with the cat on the other side of the barrier, also with some special tidbits. Lay a "Hansel and Gretel" trail of tidbits from the cat's position to the barrier in order to encourage her to approach the puppy. Keep the puppy relatively calm using the tidbits. The puppy can be encouraged to "sit" and "down" by holding the food just above his head (as the head goes up, the rear goes down) then slowly moving the food straight down to the floor and then forward. Practice these procedures for several minutes or until both animals are calm, even though they may be curious about each other. Allow them to touch noses through the barricade if they wish.

Step 3

Next, try walking the puppy around the house on a leash. Encourage the cat to stay in the vicinity by making "good things" happen to her: offer her some tidbits, play with her favorite toy, or merely hold her in your lap if she enjoys being petted. An important goal is for both animals to have pleasant things happen to them when they are in each other's presence. If neither animal is overly upset or excited, drop the puppy's leash and let him approach the cat.

Step 4

It's okay to let the cat set her own limits as to what she will tolerate from the puppy. Most puppies get the message that they have overstepped the cat's tolerance limits after several hisses and swats. Even declawed cats can intimidate a puppy. It is unlikely that a puppy will be injured by these threatening behaviors. Although a few of these limit-setting interactions are okay, don't let them become a habit. If your cat is hissing and swatting or running away every time the puppy approaches her, you need to work more on controlling their interactions as described above.

Precautions

Dogs like to eat cat food because it is very high in protein, and therefore very tasty. You should keep the cat food out of the puppy's reach (in a closet, on a high shelf, etc.) Why dogs like to "raid the litter box" is not well understood, but eating cat feces is a relatively common behavior. Although there are no health hazards to the puppy from this habit, it is usually distasteful to owners. Unfortunately, attempts to keep the puppy out of the litter box by booby trapping it will also keep the cat away as well. Punishment after the fact will *not* change the puppy's behavior. Probably the best solution is to place the litter box where the puppy cannot access it—behind a baby gate or in a closet with the door anchored open (from both sides) just wide enough for the cat, for example.

If even after following these introduction procedures your puppy and cat are not getting along, ask your veterinarian for more information or for a referral to a behavior specialist. The certified applied animal behaviorists at Animal Behavior Associates, Inc., will be happy to consult with you and help you work with your pets.

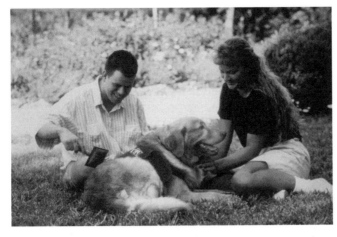

Courtesy of Frank
Siteman and
Delta Society.

Appendix H

Puppy Survival Manual: "It's a Dog's Life"

LIFE MAP for: _____*(pet's name)*

The *primary* role this dog will play in my life is:

    Member of the family
    Protection
    Breeding animal
    Show dog
    Playmate for my children
    Working dog: job description:
    Other:

This dog will live: Outside Inside Both

Other pets in the household:

This dog will spend an average of _____ hours alone each day.

The sample "life map" in this appendix is provided courtesy of Carriage Hills Animal Clinic, Montgomery, AL.

Health Protection:

Age	Vaccinations	Fecal Exam
6 wks.	DA2PL and Parvo	Yes
9 wks.	DA2PL and Parvo	Yes
12 wks.	DA2PL and Parvo	Yes
16 wks.	DA2PL, Parvo, and Rabies	Yes
20 wks.	DA2PL, Parvo, and Bordetella	No
Annually	DA2PL, Parvo, Rabies and Bordetella	Yes/HW
Semi-annually	(Vaccinations as needed)	Yes

Routine Physical Examinations: _____Annually   _____Semi-annually

Parasite Prevention:

ASAP Heartworm medication   _____Flea Control   _____Tick Control

Dental Care:

Home Care: _____Brushing   _____Dental Exercise

Ages to screen for professional care: every six months

Nutritional Plan:

Age for:

_____Growth nutrition:_____

_____Adult maintenance:_____

_____Stress management:_____
(Working years, gestation and lactation, convalescence, weight control)

Elective Procedures (Best Time):

12–14 wks.	Cosmetic ear trim
_____	Pet identification system (microchip/tag/tattoo)
6 mos.	Diagnostic Radiographs (Penn Hip) of hips for dogs over 40 pounds
6 mos.	Ovariohysterectomy (early neuter programs are available)
9 mos.	Castration (early neuter programs are available)
Annually	Lead II cardiac screen
Annually	Glaucoma screen (e.g., for certain breeds, Ton-o-pen)
_____	Breeding—provided screening tests for breed soundness are in order:
_____	OFA and/or other orthopedic clearances
	_____CERF _____VWD _____SAS

Elective Procedures (Best Time): *(cont'd)*

_____	Prebreeding evaluations:
_____	Brucellosis test
_____	Physical exam/cytology
_____	Postwhelping physical for dam and puppies
6 yrs.	"Over 40" physicals
	CBC (complete blood chemistry)—retested annually
_____	Urinalysis—retested annually
_____	Blood chemistry profiles—retested annually
_____	Electrocardiogram
_____	Screen thoracic radiographs
_____	Screening abdominal radiographs

Education:
Best time for:

	New Puppy Seminar
ASAP	(For owners with puppies under 5 mos. of age)
	Adult Basic Obedience Class
_____	(Anytime after 5 mos. of age)
	Graduate Studies
_____	(Conformation: 8 wks./Field: 8 wks./ Protection: 18 mos.)

Grooming:
How Often? (**D**aily, **W**eekly, **M**onthly)

_____Bath
_____Comb/brush
_____Clean ears
_____Trim nails
_____Brush teeth
_____Professional grooming

Behavior Management Resources: (Areas in which you would like additional assistance.)

_____Pet environmental management
_____Sharpening communication skills with your pet
_____Disciplinary techniques
_____Behavior modification and problem solving
_____Breeding, whelping, and puppy rearing guidance
_____Community outreach programs—possibilities for you and your dog
_____School programs/resource materials
_____Training programs
_____Special needs:

The Golden Years (Life expectancy for this breed: _____ years):

8 + yrs.   Senior friends examination and evaluation (CBC, blood chemistry profile, urinalysis, EKG, chest x-rays)

_____   Environmental changes (i.e., sleeping arrangements, confinement, diet and exercise, grooming)

_____   Preparation for "rainbow bridge"

• Pain versus suffering discussion
• Life extending healthcare options

We know how much you care!

NEW PET: SUPPLY CHECK LIST
(• Basic Necessities)

Nutrition:
• Recommended food: ———————————————————————
Supplements: _____

• Stainless steel food and water bowls

Parasite Prevention:
• Heartworm prevention: _____
Flea control: _____

Environment Control:
• Dog crate
Pet gate
Bitter Apple spray/cream
Flea control products: _____

Training Supplies:
• Six-foot training leash
• Web/leather collar
(Choke collar for dogs that are six months or older)
Treats

Grooming Supplies:
(Flea) shampoo: _____
Brush
Comb
Dental supplies: _____
Nail clippers
Other _____

Toys: (Variety of textures and shapes)
• Ball
Squeaky Toy
Soft Toy
• Chew Bone
Rawhides

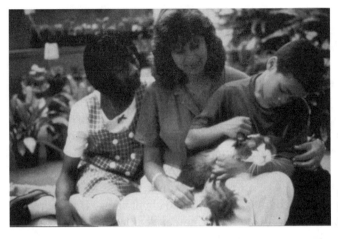

Courtesy of Frank
Siteman and
Delta Society.

Appendix I

Purr-fect Time for Cat Practices

Dogs have owners or stewards, but cats have people who wait on them.
—Observation of Reality

A HUMAN'S BEST friend may be the dog, but it appears that cats have replaced diamonds as a woman's best friend. The domestic cat population has increased steadily and in 1989 they finally outnumbered our canine companions. The better news is that according to the 1991 and 1995 AVMA Charles Charles and Associates demographic update, and subsequent reports from the AVMA and Pet Food Institute, felines have also increased their annual visits to veterinarians; over 65 percent report seeing their veterinarian annually.

Your Practice Demographics

Current U.S. data says that about 40 percent of dog households have cats, that "cat only" households average 2.5 felines, and that the 60 percent of American family units have pets (1.6 pets per household). I challenge you to evaluate 100 consecutive medical records in your files and compare your own practice demographics to these figures.

The science of demographics makes veterinary marketing a little easier. For instance, *American Demographics* recently published data indicating that Portland,

Oregon, has the highest demand for dry cat food. For a practitioner in that city, it would be wise to target this market by highlighting feline nutritional counseling as well as the premium diets available through the veterinary practice. Depending on personal comfort zones, this could be a client newsletter, a target mailing to cat owners on a postcard, or even a coupon system in a local media source.

What if you are not in Portland, Oregon, or do not have that comfort zone for target mailings. Your own practice demographics can still tell you if you are asking the right questions of your clients. Do you ask about other pets when a new client accesses the practice? Are all the pet records in a single household screened by the receptionist each time an established client visits? Has the receptionist staff been empowered to discuss routine pet healthcare needs with the client, by saying something like, "I noticed your kitty appears past due for some protective vaccinations. I have made a note in the medical records so that the Doctor will remember to talk to you about it." Try some of these ideas routinely for 90 days, then screen another 100 records. Most practices will be surprised by the difference the receptionist's concern makes in gross and return visits.

Marketing to the Feline Owner

Marketing is not always comfortable, but it is not always advertising either. Walk into your own reception room, stop, and look around. Is the room "dog heavy" with pictures and books, or is there a balance between cat and dog graphics? Can cat owners sit away from massive canines that look like they would swallow a cat whole? Does the reception area offer a Plexiglass holding box with a white rug and clear lid for unruly or nervous cats? Pick up your hospital brochure and see if your practice is feline friendly, in word or by picture. Move to the exam room and review the image the walls give. Are the exam tables built low for large dogs or have certain rooms been raised for cats? Is there a cat examination room? Do the routine handouts balance dog needs with cat needs?

If you are deeper into marketing, look at the yellow pages in your community. How many people have targeted the growing feline market? A simple listing that reflects special cat healthcare hours without dogs present, special feline boarding facilities, or cat bathing/healthcare supplies may be all it takes to differentiate your practice. These same features could be just published in a special tri-fold, low cost, feline brochure available at the front counter.

Many practices are starting to stock "impulse buy" items near their discharge counter. Look at your discharge area. Is it for dog owners or cat owners? Many cat owners are looking for that real catnip, a good way of watering their multi-cat household, or even an escape proof carrier.

The Competitive Edge

In today's veterinary marketplace, there is competition, not only from our colleagues, but also from drug stores, pet shops, and those emerging mass market animal food stores. They all want our clients to come to them. In marketing we are taught to do the unusual as if it were usual or to do the usual as if it were unusual. Most practices have a slow mid-day period, so why not target that in an unusual manner, such as "exclusive time for feline healthcare appointments." An example of the unusual as usual could be simply joining cages by a small door and marketing them as cat condos (extra cage space for an additional fee in times of low occupancy). This reverse approach has proven profitable in more than one boarding complex.

It is the responsibility of each practice to target those clients they want to attract and retain. I am surprised at the number of good practices that complain about their client mix. They do not realize that their clients are exactly the ones they have developed over the years. A practice starts to develop its own client mix after the first few months of operation. Each practice should have a written plan showing where they want the client mix to go during the next six months, the next year, and the next three years, and how they plan to achieve that goal. Does each staff member know their role in making the goal happen?

Becoming Feline Friendly

This is a practice philosophy decision, so let's just assume from the above discussion that you want more cat clients. First, the examination room for cats needs to be a "cat room"; if there is a window ledge, so much the better. Have cat pictures and cat resources in this room, and it can be "more cozy" than a dog room, which means fewer square feet. Have the cat ward away from the dog ward and have it clearly marked so clients believe that you believe in the segregation.

For boarding dogs, we have always seen runs as a special benefit. We have even sold them at higher fees. We also have seen "play time" enter the canine boarding market. What is the equivalent for cats in your care?

- *Cat condos.* Many cage manufacturers have established cat condos, which allow vertical or horizontal movement between cage units. This allows the cat owner to purchase more "rooms" for kitty, and it allows the practice to realize a greater net during nonpeak boarding times. The second "room" is generally offered at a reduced rate to the standard "cage fee."
- *Feline habitats.* This concept was first called a "cat closet," more as a descriptive term than as a client bonding phrase. We call them "habitats" and offer play time in them for an additional fee. At one practice, small three- to four-foot runs have been converted to habitats; each has been painted as a "vacation land" such as Disney, Tahiti, New Orleans, Las Vegas, etc., and "twice-a-day kitty vacations" are being offered to cat owners who board their cats. Some have asked to lease the vacation land full time for their kitty, and for $18-plus a day, the practice does allow this.
- *"Cages."* New cage units (such as the white injection molded units) have come on the market that can be "back lit" by fluorescent tubes so the "cave syndrome" becomes history. Also, changing the doors from bars to clear Plexiglass makes the units very client friendly. This has also occurred with dog cages. Using

small wall-light sconces, chandeliers, brass beds, framed pictures screwed to the cage wall, and other accessories makes these "glass door" units really seem like up-scale bedroom units. The practices which pursue the "no bar" boarding units charge above the community top dollar, and they all have waiting lists.

• *Play time.* For practices without habitats or condos, allowing the cat out of the cage to freely roam in the ward has been tried, but you must ensure FeLV, FIV, FIP, and vaccination status on *all feline boarders* then!

Many of your feline owners worry about "locking kitty away" for a period of time. How much your practice can excite clients about the "environment" kitty will be in can cause greater client satisfaction and greater practice liquidity. Cats are quieter and cleaner than dogs, and they have teeth and claws that, while dangerous, need veterinary care. One animal caretaker can generally support 32 dogs in an eight-hour shift, but the same person can support over 45 cats in the same time. So don't just sit there, make a decision about what you want to do and get the practice team to understand "why" you want to do it, now!

Empowering Your Staff

We are all well aware that the veterinarian produces the gross, but we often forget that it is the staff who makes the net happen. The staff of any practice is the difference between success and frustration. Ask your staff what the three primary practice goals are for this year. If their answers do not agree, you have found one of your problems. As you develop a feline practice philosophy, make the objectives very clear to the staff and empower them to make it happen. Allow them to talk cats with clients or go to local cat shows and talk with breeders and exhibitors. That is how a staff can make the difference in developing your feline practice.

If you are brave, ask a staff member, "How's your number one?" In the best of cases, they should reply with one of the practice core values, with one of the practice's short-term objectives, or with one of their performance plan targets for this quarter (but that is another leadership topic altogether). In most practices, the staff members just stumble and stammer. In program-based budgeting, the new service or new product is a new income center. The new program only works if the practice staff believes in the "why" of the effort. They must be proud of the new program or new service. Some of the ideas shared above, such as no bars on the cage doors, cat habitats, or representing the practice at a cat show, will make most any staff member proud. It has been shown in human healthcare that when pride is the input by the staff, the client perceives quality as the output of the healthcare encounter. This is the magic competitive edge that bonds a client to the practice, and the ideas shared above are targeted to bond the "cat person" to the practice. Now make the staff believe in the "why" and stand back. Magic will occur.

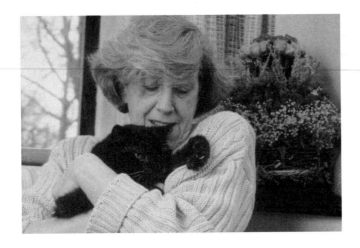

Appendix J

Information for the New Cat Owner

THE MATERIAL in this appendix represents a series of handouts for new and prospective cat owners.

So You Want a Cat? Some Things for Prospective Cat Owners to Think About

Bringing a cat into your home is a wonderful experience but it is also a serious responsibility. Below are some questions, for you and your family members to ask yourselves about your own needs and your expectations of the cat, that will help you pick out the pet best suited to you. Try to be as realistic and honest as possible in answering these questions.

1. Why do you want a cat?

What do you expect the cat to do? Will she just be a companion for you? Will she be a companion for your children? Do you expect her to hunt mice or rats? Different breeds or individuals within a breed may be better suited to some roles than to others.

Special recognition for these contributions goes to Daniel O. Estep, Ph.D., and Suzanne Hetts, Ph.D., Animal Behavior Associates, Inc., 4994 S. Independence Way, Littleton, CO 80123, (303) 932-9095.

2. What's your family like now? What do you expect it to be in 5 to 10 years?

Are you single, married, or married with children, and do you have older relatives in the home? Are you single now but expect to start a family soon? Your choice of pet should take into account not only your present family status but also your expected future status. A cat chosen for a single person may not be suited for a family with children. Remember that owning a pet is a lifetime commitment.

3. What is your home like? Do you want your cat to be an inside cat, outside cat, or both?

Do you live in a small apartment, house with a fenced yard, etc.? Letting your cat outside exposes her to certain risks such as injuries from cars, cat fights, and other animals. Are you prepared to live with those risks?

4. What pets do you already have? Are you planning on having other pets in the near future besides the cat?

Many cats don't get along well with other animals (and vice versa). You should think very carefully before bringing a new cat into a household with other pets that she may not get along with.

5. What is your lifestyle like?

Are you very active and rarely home, fairly inactive and home most of the time, or somewhere in between? Do you have activities that you want your cat to be a part of? Cats are social animals and need some companionship; however, some cats may tolerate more isolation than others. If you are very active and rarely home perhaps you should consider another kind of pet.

6. What temperament do you want in your cat?

Do you want a very active cat or very inactive cat? Do you want one that is shy or very outgoing with strangers? What about a cat that demands a lot of attention? A cat's temperament is very important to how well it will fit into your household. You should consider very carefully what temperament characteristics you want in your cat and then consult with your veterinarian, breeders, and other animal experts about the best cat for you. When picking a cat, never pick one that seems fearful, aggressive, or overly active.

7. What breed of cat do you want? Why?

Do you want a purebred cat or a mixed breed cat? Never pick a cat solely on its looks or its physical characteristics. It may not have the temperament or other characteristics you want. Consult books, breeders, your veterinarian, and friends who own a breed you are considering to help choose a breed. Consider a mixed breed cat from a shelter. They often have fewer physical and behavioral problems than do purebred cats, but may be more of a gamble with an unknown history. If you buy a purebred cat, only buy from an established breeder with a good reputation.

8. What kind of coat characteristics and coat color do you want?

Some coats are more likely to shed and tangle than others and will require more care.

9. What sex cat do you want? Why?

Each sex has its own advantages and disadvantages, special needs and problems. Males are more likely to roam, urine mark, and fight with other cats, for example. All cats should be spayed or neutered unless you are planning to show the cat competitively or breed the cat. Spaying and neutering reduces the chances of certain behavioral and medical problems as well as reducing the pet over-population problem.

10. What age cat do you want? Why?

Kittens can be lots of fun, but they can be a lot of work to housebreak, train to a scratching post, and socialize. Are you prepared to put in the work necessary to have a kitten?

11. Have you thought through the potential costs and problems associated with owning a cat?

Owning a cat can be a very rich and rewarding experience. However along with the rewards come problems and costs. There will be a time commitment required; feeding, grooming, and healthcare costs; cleaning up after the cat; and some destruction of your property by the cat. Are you committed to dealing with these problems and costs? Remember that owning a cat is a lifetime commitment.

Preventing Aggressive Behavior by Kittens

Aggression by cats directed at people is *the* most serious problem faced by owners. Aggressive cats can cause serious injury. There is nothing that an owner can do that will absolutely guarantee that a kitten will never become aggressive. This is because our knowledge about the causes of aggression is incomplete. However, there are some things that you can do as an owner that will lessen the likelihood that your kitten will become aggressive. Some of these things are designed to prevent kitten aggression, while others are designed to prevent aggression as your cat grows up.

Genetics and Breeding

Genetics and breeding can influence aggression and other problem behaviors.

- If you buy a kitten, purchase it from an established breeder with a good reputation. Always ask the breeder about the parents and brothers and sisters of the kitten. Never buy a kitten whose parents or siblings have been aggressive or fearful of people. Be sure that the kitten has had plenty of contact with people and other cats. Avoid buying kittens that seem overly excitable or overly fearful.
- If you get a cat from a shelter or pet store where you cannot ask about the parents or siblings, don't pick a cat that is overly excitable or overly fearful. Avoid getting a cat that has been living by itself with little contact with other cats or people.

Out of Control Play

Out of control play is one of the most common causes of injury by kittens. Kittens should always be encouraged to play gently with people.
- *Never* encourage a kitten to play roughly and to bite or mouth clothing or skin. This only rewards unacceptable behavior. Children should be taught acceptable ways to play with kittens and supervised to be sure that they are not encouraging bad behavior.

- If the kitten tries to bite, nip, or play roughly, (1) try to direct her play onto a ball, string, or other appropriate toy, (2) put the kitten on a time-out for a few minutes away from people, or (3) use remote punishment to discourage rough play. Remote punishment means telling the kitten "no" at the same time you squirt her with water or make a loud, startling sound like shaking a can full of pennies. The punishment should always occur during the rough play, never after. If you cannot catch her in the act, don't punish her. *Never* hit, slap, kick, or use other physical punishment with a kitten. It is unnecessary and may make the problem worse.
- Always try to make touching, petting, and grooming the kitten a calm, relaxed, nonplayful situation. Encouraging play in these situations will only make it more difficult for the kitten to learn the difference between play and nonplay situations.

Fear and Pain

Fear and pain are the other major causes of kittens injuring people.

- *Never* hit, slap, kick, or hurt a kitten. It is cruel and may cause the kitten to bite or become fearful of you.
- Young children should never be left alone with kittens or allowed to hurt or scare them.
- Never scare kittens with loud noises, sudden movements, or other frightening events.
- If your kitten is frightened of sounds, things (like vacuum cleaners), or people, get professional help.
- Kittens should be taught to tolerate handling; being restrained, petted, groomed, and moved around; and having food and toys taken from them. Rewards, *not force* should be used to get the kitten to comply so that she has a good attitude about these things. These activities should be done regularly as a normal part of play, feeding, grooming, etc.
- Simple rules should be developed by the family as to what the kitten can and can't do around the house (such as getting on the furniture, getting food scraps from the table, going outside, etc.). These rules should be enforced consistently by all family members.
- Punishment for misbehavior of any sort should be done only when other things have been tried and have failed. Punishment should only be of the remote kind: a loud noise, water squirted on the kitten, or a small pillow thrown in the general direction of the kitten (*don't* hit the kitten with the pillow).

Territorial and Protective Aggression

Territorial and protective aggression occurs when a cat tries to drive away unfamiliar people or cats from her territory or from people or cats she is attached to.

- Neutering male cats and spaying female cats may reduce the likelihood of territorial or possessive aggression developing.
- Kittens should be socialized with other cats and unfamiliar people. This means gradual, nonthreatening exposure associated with rewards (food, play, petting) while your cat is nonaggressive, nonfearful, relaxed, and comfortable.
- Kittens should be taught to be calm and quiet when people or cats pass by your

property (including your car), come on your property, or come into your house. Use food or other rewards to get your cat to sit or lie down quietly.

• Physical punishment should not be used to stop cats that are growling, threatening, or out of control around unfamiliar people or dogs.

Redirected Agression

Redirected aggression occurs when a cat is strongly motivated to aggress against another person or animal but is prevented from doing so.

• Never break up a fight between two cats with your hands or other parts of your body. One or both cats may turn and attack you.
• Never touch, pet, or try to hold a cat that is hissing, growling, or meowing aggressively at another cat or person.
• A cat can remain aggressive *for over an hour* after becoming aggressive. Be very cautious about approaching, touching, or handling a cat you know has been aggressive within the last hour or so.

Predatory Behavior

Predatory behavior occurs when cats attempt to hunt and kill small animals like squirrels or birds.

• Kittens should never be encouraged to hunt small animals or birds or to excitedly chase any animal or person.
• Kittens caught in the act of stalking, chasing, or lunging at people or other animals should be discouraged by loudly approaching them, making a loud sound, or squirting them with water.
• Kittens should never be punished after the fact for stalking, chasing, or lunging or for carrying or consuming prey.
• Restrict the kitten's access to small animals and birds to prevent predation.

Get Professional Help

If an aggression problem develops, get professional help immediately, do not wait. It is very likely that the longer you wait, the worse the problem will become.

If you find yourself punishing your cat more than just occasionally, seek professional help to deal with the problem.

Preventing Damage Due to Kitten Scratching

The first thing you should know is that scratching by kittens is a perfectly natural, normal behavior. It is unlikely that anything you do will stop it completely. What we will try to do is give you some things to do to lessen the damage. You should accept the fact that if you own a cat you will experience property damage and lose something of value. The basic strategies in preventing kitten damage, are to (1) prevent access to things that you don't want damaged or to make those things give the animal an unpleasant experience when they try to damage it and (2) provide acceptable things to scratch.

Scratching or clawing objects with the front paws is mainly a social marking behavior to let other cats and people know the cat is around. It is only secondarily that it aids in keeping the claws sharp. The location and texture of the surface to be scratched is very important to the cat.

- Most kittens prefer a vertical scratching post, some like a horizontal post. Provide both initially to see which one your cat prefers.
- Cats like to scratch soon after getting up after sleeping, and to mark prominent areas in their chief activity areas. Place scratching posts near sleep spots and near couches, chairs, and/or doorways where the cat is most active. Put out at least three or four posts around the house.
- Cats generally prefer posts with a covering that is easily shredded. If your post covering is not of this type, cover the post with a loose weave fabric or other material that is easily shredded. Don't replace the covering too soon. Cats like the material very worn. Wait until it is just about to fall off the post before replacing it.
- Encourage your cat to scratch on the posts. Dont take the kitten to the post and forcibly drag its claws over the post. This will only make the cat afraid of you and the post. Lure the cat to the post with a string or dangle toy and encourage the cat to scratch the post as it plays. Reward the cat with praise and/or food treats whenever it scratches the post.
- *Never* use physical punishment when your kitten scratches an inappropriate object. Gently take the cat to its post and encourage her to scratch it. If this is not possible, make a loud sound like dropping a book or squirt her with water from a water bottle. *Never* punish a kitten for scratching things if you don't catch her in the act.
- Observe your kitten's scratching behavior carefully to see where and what surfaces she prefers to scratch. Use this information to place posts in your kitten's most preferred areas and to cover posts with the most preferred coverings.
- Seek professional help if your kitten won't use her post or if you are having trouble implementing these suggestions.

Remember: An ounce of prevention is worth a pound of cure. It is far easier to establish good habits from the beginning than to break bad habits later.

Introducing Your New Kitten to Your Other Cats

Most species of cats, including the domestic house cat, are basically solitary. They do not form highly structured social groups with the same types of social hierarchies or "pecking orders" as do dogs. Although cats *can* form close attachments to other animals, they are also very territorial. There is wide individual variation in how tolerant individual cats are of sharing their house and territory with multiple cats.

How Will the Resident Cat Accept a New Kitten?

The factors which determine how a resident cat(s) will accept a newcomer are not fully understood. Cats who are well socialized, meaning they had many pleasant experiences with other cats during kittenhood, will likely be more sociable than cats who did not. Stray cats who were "street cats" and were in the habit of fighting with other cats in order to defend their territory and food resources may not do as well in a multi-cat household. If the resident cats have been in the habit of chasing intruding cats off their territory or growling at neighborhood cats through the window, they may have a more difficult time accepting a newcomer.

Genetic factors also influence a cat's temperament, so friendly parents, especially friendly fathers, may be more likely to produce friendly offspring.

A new kitten well may want to play with the older resident cat or may be somewhat fearful of him. Kittens are unlikely to show territorial or inter-male aggression as do adult cats. The resident cat may either respond in a playful manner or show defensive, inter-male, or territorial aggression.

Cats who live in the same house may become the best of friends, or they may only tolerate each other with a minimum of conflict. However, there will be some individual cats who are better off in single-cat households. The initial interactions a newcomer and resident cat have can "set the stage" for their future relationship. It is much better to introduce cats to each other very gradually, over a period of several weeks or even months, if necessary, than to start off with an aggressive encounter which could take even longer to overcome.

Introducing a New Kitten to a Resident Family Cat

Step 1

Confine the kitten to one medium sized room with her litter box, toys, scratching post, food, water, and a bed. Feed the resident cat and the newcomer near either side of the door to this room. Depending on your feeding schedule, this can either be the cats' regular meals or special "goodies" they will get only as part of the introduction process. This will help to start things out on the right foot by associating something enjoyable (eating!) with each other's presence. Don't put the food so close to the door that the cats are too upset by each other's presence to eat. Gradually move the dishes closer to the door until the cats can eat *calmly* directly on either side. Next, use two doorstops to prop open the door just enough to allow the cats to see each other, and repeat the whole process.

Step 2

Switch sleeping blankets between the kitten and resident cat so they have a chance to become accustomed to each other's scent. Also put the scented blankets underneath the food dishes.

Step 3

Spend some quiet time in the kitten's room. Sit down on the floor or the bed and let the kitten approach you. Don't stare at her, and scratch her gently under the chin or behind the ears. Before you go into her room, take a few minutes to pet the resident cat so you have his scent. Take some tidbits and/or a dangling toy with you so that the kitten associates you and the scent of the other cat with "good things."

Step 4

Once the kitten is using her litter box, eating regularly, approaching the door without fear or aggression while the resident cat is on the other side, and is comfortable with your presence in her room, let her have some free time in the house while putting the resident cat in the kitten's room. This switch provides another way for the cats to have experience with each other's scent without a face-to-face meeting and also allows the kitten to become familiar with her new surroundings without being frightened by the resident cat.

Step 5

After several of these switches, if both cats are becoming less curious about each other's scents and things have been going well on either side of the closed door during feeding or "treat" times, then it's time for a brief face-to-face introduction. There are a variety of ways to do this, depending on the cats and the physical environment. If either cat is used to and comfortable in a crate, one or both of them can be crated. Cover the crate(s) with a towel and allow only one side open so the cats don't feel so exposed. Do *not* use a crate if this will be the cat's first experience with one or if the cat is not calm while crated. If both cats are crated, the crates can gradually be moved closer to each other. Food treats should be offered to both. If one cat is loose, let this cat approach the crate at her own speed. Alternatively, one or both cats can be held on the owners' laps (if the cats enjoy this). Do not force the cats to stay there if they become excited—this could result in someone being bitten or scratched. Use food treats and allow the cats to approach each other on their own.

With either method, keep the interaction short, and end it while both cats are still curious and/or calm, not aggressive or fearful. Repeat this process, making each session a little longer if things are going well. In the meantime, continue to keep the cats separated.

This stage in the introduction process may be reached in several days, or it may take several weeks. How well the cats are responding to each other will determine when it's time to move ahead—there is no one correct time schedule.

Step 6

Avoid any interactions between the cats which result in either fearful or aggressive behavior. If this happens during a face-to-face introduction, calmly separate the cats and continue the introduction process using the gradual steps outlined above. You may need to find another intermediate step to work with before the cats will be ready for another try at a face-to face interaction. *Never put two cats together and allow them to "fight it out."* If these responses are allowed to become a habit, they can be difficult to change.

Precautions: You'll need to add another litter box and probably clean all the boxes more frequently. Make sure that none of the cats is being "ambushed" by another while trying to use the box.

Try to keep the resident cat's schedule as close as possible to what it was before the kitten's appearance.

If problems persist or arise, consult your veterinarian for more information or for a referral to a behavior specialist. The certified applied animal behaviorists at Animal Behavior Associates, Inc., will be happy to consult with you and help you work with your pets.

Introducing Your New Kitten to Your Dog

Dogs and cats who were not exposed to each other's species when they were young will require some extra time to become accustomed to each other. An adult dog will most likely consider a kitten to be either a plaything or prey and consequently will either want to play with it or harm it. A kitten may be very intimidated by an adult dog. Dogs and cats will react to each other differently because they differ in their communication signals and social behaviors. They will need to be introduced to each other slowly and gradually so that neither is harmed or frightened and aggressive reactions don't become a habit.

Introducing a Kitten to a Resident Dog

Step 1

If your dog does not already know the commands "sit," "down," "come," and "stay," you should begin working on them. Little tidbits of food increase your dog's motivation to perform, which will be necessary in the presence of such a strong distraction as a new kitten! Even if your dog already knows the commands, work with obeying commands in return for a tidbit so that your dog will perform more willingly and reliably.

Step 2

When you first bring her home, confine the kitten to one medium-sized room with her litter box, toys, scratching post, food, water, and a bed. Feed the dog and the kitten near either side of the door to this room. Depending on your feeding schedule, this can either be the animals' regular meals or special "goodies" they will get only as part of the introduction process. This will help to start things out on the right foot by associating something enjoyable (eating) with each other's presence. Don't put the food so close to the door that either the dog or the kitten are too upset or distracted by each other's presence to eat. Gradually move the dishes closer to the door until the animals can eat calmly directly on either side. Next, use two doorstops to prop open the door just enough—maybe only an inch—to allow the animals to see each other, and repeat the whole process.

Step 3

Switch sleeping blankets between the kitten and dog so they have a chance to become accustomed to each other's scent. Also put the scented blankets underneath the food dishes.

Step 4

Spend some quiet time in the kitten's room. Sit down on the floor or the bed and let the kitten approach you. Don't stare at her, and scratch her gently under the chin or behind the ears. Before you go in her room, take a few minutes to pet the dog so you have his scent. Take some tidbits and/or a dangling toy with you so that the kitten associates you and the scent of the dog with "good things."

Step 5

Once the kitten is using her litter box, eating regularly, approaching the door without fear or aggression while the dog is on the other side, and is comfortable with your presence in her room, let her have some free time in the house while putting the dog in the kitten's room. This switch provides another way for the animals to have experience with each other's scent without a face-to-face meeting and also allows the kitten to become familiar with her new surroundings without being frightened by the dog.

Step 6

After several of these switches, if the animals are becoming less curious about each other's scents and things have been going well on either side of the closed door during feeding or "treat" times, then it's time for a brief face-to-face introduction. Put your dog's leash on and command him to either "sit" or "down" and "stay," using food tidbits. Have another family member enter the room and quietly sit down with the kitten on his/her lap. The kitten should also be offered some special tidbits. If the kitten does not like to be held, you can use a wire crate or carrier instead if the kitten is used to and comfortable in a crate. Cover the crate with a towel and allow only one side open so the kitten doesn't feel so exposed. Do not use a crate if this will be the kitten's first experience with one or if the kitten is not calm while crated. At first, the kitten and dog should be on *opposite* sides of the room or as far apart as necessary so that neither becomes fearful, aggressive, or out of control. Repeat this step several times until both are relatively calm and just curious about each other. Do not progress to the next step until this has happened. This may take several days or more of practice.

Step 7

Next, move the animals a little closer together, with the dog still on leash and the kitten either held gently in a lap or crated. If the dog gets up from his "stay" position, he should be firmly repositioned, praised, and given a tidbit for obeying the "stay" command. If the kitten becomes frightened, increase the distance between the animals and progress more slowly. Eventually, the animals should be brought close enough together to allow them to investigate each other. If the kitten is not frightened and wants to walk toward the dog on her own, let her do so as long as the dog remains under control.

Step 8

When the kitten and the dog can be calm when close to each other, you can begin letting each move around a little more in the other's presence. Continue to keep the dog in a "down-stay" using tidbits and let the kitten explore the room. If she's still a little timid, you can encourage her with a toy. Then switch roles: hold or crate the kitten and let the dog walk around. Keep the dog on leash, even in a heel position if he is still quite excited. If he is doing well, let him approach the kitten on his own. With each practice session, increase the time the animals spend together and gradually let them have more freedom of movement. Be sure that your cat has an escape route and a place to hide. Keep the dog and cat separated when you aren't home until you are certain the cat will be safe.

Step 9

Avoid any interactions between the animals which result in either fearful or aggressive behavior. If this happens during a face-to-face introduction, calmly separate them and continue the introduction process using the gradual steps outlined above. You may need to find another intermediate step to practice before allowing the same amount of contact again.

Developing successful relationships between cats and dogs can require a lot of time and patience. Sometimes the two can become best of friends, while other times they only develop a mutual respect and tolerance of one another. If you have problems, ask your veterinarian for more information or for a referral to a behavior specialist. The certified applied animal behaviorists at Animal Behavior Associates, Inc., will be happy to consult with you and help you work with your pets.

Your New Cat and the Litter Box—Preventing Problems

When a kitten is about four weeks of age, she/he will begin to play in, explore, and dig in loose, soft materials, such as dirt or litter. Soon, this investigative digging results in the kitten eliminating in these materials. Many species of cats begin to show this behavior as soon as they can eliminate on their own. Kittens do not have to be taught by either their mothers or their human owners to relieve themselves in soft, loose materials or to dig and bury their waste. These behaviors are called "innate" behaviors because kittens do not have to learn how to perform them. However, where a cat eliminates can be affected by its experiences. Litter boxes that for a variety of possible reasons do not provide an acceptable place to eliminate *from the cat's point of view,* may cause a cat to go to the bathroom somewhere else. Thus, it is important for you to provide a litter box which meets your new kitten's or cat's needs so that she/he will like the box and use it consistently.

The Myth of "Litter-Training" Cats

There is really no such thing as "litter-training" a cat in the same way one would house train a dog. The only thing owners need to do is provide an acceptable, accessible litter box, using the criteria described below. Remember that what is acceptable and accessible must be determined from the cat's point of view, not the owner's. It is not necessary, or even recommended, to take a cat to the box and move his paws back and forth in the litter. This may actually be an unpleasant experience for the cat and may initiate "bad" associations with the litter box. As explained above, a cat does not need to be taught what to do with a litter box. If you provide him with acceptable, accessible litter, he'll know what it's for.

Choosing a Location for the Box

Most cat owners want to place the litter box in an out-of-the-way place in order to minimize odor and loose particles of cat litter tracked around the house. Often, the litter box may end up in the basement, possibly next to an appliance, on an unfinished, cold cement floor. This type of location may be undesirable from the cat's point of view. First, if you have a young, small kitten, she/he may not be able to get down a long flight of steep stairs in time when she/he has to go to the bathroom—especially if she/he started out on the top floor of a multi-level home. Even adult cats new to a household may not at first remember where the box is located if it is in an area they seldom frequent. Secondly, cats may be startled while using the box if a furnace or washer/dryer suddenly comes on. That may be the last time they'll risk such a frightening experience! Lastly, some cats like to scratch the surface surrounding their litter box and may find a cold cement floor unappealing. So you may have to compromise. The box should be kept in a location which affords the cat some privacy, but is also conveniently located. If you place the box in a closet, be sure the door is wedged open from both sides in order to prevent your cat from being trapped in or out. If the box sits on a smooth, slick or cold surface, consider putting a small throw rug underneath the box.

Choosing a Litter

Research has shown that most cats prefer fine-grained litters, presumably because they have a softer feel. The new clumping litters are usually finer grained than the typical clay litter. However, high quality, dust-free clay litters are relatively small grained and may be perfectly acceptable. Potting soil also has a very soft texture but is not very absorbent. If you suspect your cat had an outdoor history or is likely to eliminate in your houseplants, you can try mixing some potting soil with your regular litter. Pellet-type litters or those made from citrus peels are not recommended. Once you find a litter your cat likes, don't change types or brands. Buying generic, the least expensive, or whatever brand is on sale may result in litter box problems.

Some cat litters were developed more with the owner's needs than the cat's needs in mind. Many cats are put off by the odor of scented or deodorant litters. For the same reason, it is not a good idea to place a room deodorizer or air freshener near the litter box. A thin layer of baking soda can be placed on the bottom of the box to help absorb odors without repelling the cat. More importantly, if the litter box is kept clean, odor should not be a problem.

Depth of Litter

Some owners are under the impression that the more litter they put in the box, the less often they will have to clean it. *Not!!* When wild cats eliminate outside, they generally choose an area that has a few loose particles of dirt or other material in which they can make a scrape. They generally *do not* choose areas where they "sink in" to several inches of dirt. Most domestic cats will not like litter that is more than about two inches deep. In fact, some cats, particularly some long-haired cats, may actually prefer less litter and a smooth, slick surface such as the bottom of the litter box. The box *must* be cleaned on a regular basis, and adding extra litter is not a way around that chore.

Number of Boxes

A good guideline is to have at least as many boxes as you have cats. That way, no cat can be prevented from using the box because it is already occupied. You might also consider placing the boxes in several locations around the house, so that no one cat can "guard" the litter box area and prevent other cats from accessing it. In general, it is not possible to designate a personal, unique box for each cat in the household. Cats will often use any and all litter boxes available. Occasionally a cat will refuse to use the box after another cat. In this case, all boxes will need to be kept extremely clean, and extra boxes may be needed.

Are Covered Boxes Better?

Many cats will not show any preference for a covered versus an uncovered box. However, if you have a very large cat, a covered box may not allow him sufficient room to turn around, scratch and dig, and position himself in the way he wants. A covered box may also make it easier for another cat to lay in wait and "ambush" the user as she/he exits the box. On the other hand, a covered box tends to provide more privacy and may be preferred by timid, shy cats. You may need to experiment and offer both types at first to discover what your cat prefers. If you do not wish to purchase a cover, you can make one from an upside-down cardboard box with the flaps and one side cut away.

Keeping the Litter Box Clean

Litter boxes must be kept consistently clean. To meet the needs of the most discriminating cat, feces should be scooped out of the box daily. How often you change the litter depends on the number of cats and the number of boxes you have. Twice a week is a general guideline, but depending on the circumstances, the litter may need to be changed every other day or only once a week. If you notice an odor to the box or if much of the litter is wet or clumped, it's probably more than time for a change.

Do not use strong smelling chemicals or cleaning products when washing the box. The smell of vinegar, bleach, or pine cleaners may cause your cat to avoid the box. Washing with soap and water should be sufficient.

What about Liners?

Some cats don't mind having a liner in the box, while others do. You may need to experiment again to see if your cat is bothered by a liner in the box. If you do use a liner, make sure it is anchored in place well so it can not easily catch your cat's claws or be pulled down into the litter.

If Problems Develop

If your cat stops using the litter box your first call should always be to your veterinarian. Many medical conditions can cause a change in litter box habits, and these possibilities must be considered first If your veterinarian determines your cat is healthy, the cause may be behavioral. Most litter box behavior problems can be resolved through behavior counseling. Both behavior modification techniques and changes to the cat's environment may be necessary. Punishment is *not* the answer. The certified applied animal behaviorists from Animal Behavior Associates, Inc., would be happy to consult with you and help you work with your cat.

Is Your Cat Stressed Out?

Stress is a word we use daily. We may use it to describe environmental events that upset us, as well as our bodies' physiological, emotional, and behavioral reactions to them. Understanding stress in other species is more difficult and confusing because we use the term imprecisely when we refer to our own species. For example, can you tell if the person sitting next to you at the movies is stressed? What if the person sitting next to you at the movies is stressed? What if the person is sitting quietly, is furiously chewing gum with an angry look on his or her face, or is visibly in pain?

Would you consider your cat to be stressed if it turned up its nose at its regular dinner, if it was being chased by your dog, or if it was lying under the bed refusing to come when called? The conclusions we draw may or may not be correct based on our interpretation of these behaviors. To better evaluate if your cat is stressed, it is helpful to have a basic understanding of what scientific research has discovered about stress.

What Is Stress?

Because stress is complex, experts find it difficult to agree on a definition. A general definition is that stress is the body's reaction to demands placed on it and an attempt to regain the body's normal balance. This reaction includes physiological and behavioral responses. The demands causing these reactions are stressors.

A brief explanation of the basic physiological stress response will help explain behaviors associated with stress. In the early part of this century, William Cannon, a physiologist who described the "fight or flight" response, and later Nans Selye, a physician who proposed the general adaptation syndrome, were the first scientists to try to better understand how animals, including humans, adapt to stressors in their environment.

When alarmed, animals mobilize their bodies' resources to prepare for action. These physiological changes include an increased heart rate, a release of sugar into the bloodstream, and increased blood flow to the internal organs. The reactions are initiated by *adrenaline,* a chemical secreted by one part (the *medulla*) of the adrenal glands, located on top of the kidneys. As this response continues or becomes prolonged, another part (the *cortex*) of the adrenal gland becomes active and secretes many hormones, including corticosteroids.

These hormones affect the body in complex ways, not all of which are well understood. They also help the body respond to stressors through their effects on the immune system, general metabolism, and other body systems. High concentrations of the corticosteroids in the blood and/or urine, particularly cortisol, are a standard criterion used to determine if stress is occurring. If large amounts of the hormones persist in reaction to chronic stressors, adverse effects can result, including decreased resistance to disease, decreased growth, gastric ulcers, decreased reproductive capabilities, and even death.

What are some examples of stressors that cause a physiological stress response? Physical stressors that wild or free-ranging animals (including feral or stray cats) often experience include disease, injury, lack of food and water, exposure to extreme weather conditions, predators, and fights with other animals. Many of these physical stressors for domesticated and captive animals have been eliminated. However, these animals are more likely to experience social or biological stressors such as social isolation, barren or restricted environments, restraint, unpredictable, unfamiliar or uncontrollable environments, or crowding that results in increased social competition and conflict.

Behavioral Responses to Stressors

Animals show behavioral responses to stressors while the physiological events previously described are taking place. Many of these behavioral responses are considered normal behaviors; these include fear or anxiety-related behaviors, aggression and related behaviors, conflict behaviors including redirected behavior, displacement behavior, approach/avoidance behavior, and separation distress. Other stress-related behaviors, such as repetitive and self-injurious behaviors, can be considered abnormal, while still others, such as refusal to eat or drink, can be associated with illness.

One of the most common stressors for cats is social conflict, which most likely occurs when a new arrival is introduced into the household or when too many cats are present in the household. Although recent studies of cat behavior have shown that cats can be flexible regarding their social structure, cats are still not considered the social animals that dogs are. While some cats in a multi-cat household will develop close, friendly relationships, others will continually harass or be harassed by other cats in the family. Both the cat being harassed and the one doing the harassing may be stressed. The harassed cat may begin hiding more and may be reluctant to move about freely. This in turn can cause changes in litter box and eating habits.

Approach/avoidance behaviors also may be common. For example, a cat may start to move across the room to lie in a favorite spot (approach) but may be scared of being discovered by the "bully" and so turns and runs the other way (avoidance). This type of rushing forward, running backward movement can become ritualized into a stereotype that is shown out of the context in which it started. Stereotypes are abnormal, repetitive behavior patterns with no apparent purpose. Tail-chasing is another stereotype seen fairly frequently in domestic cats.

Displacement behavior may appear during social conflicts. A harassed cat may be undecided about whether to run from its attacker or stand and fight. Instead, the cat displays a third, unrelated behavior, such as grooming, which is known as displacement behavior. Displacement behaviors can also evolve into stereotypes. In the case of grooming, it can become excessive to the point of causing hair loss and skin lesions.

Redirected behavior often occurs in multi-cat households in which conflicts between cats are common. Cats often direct aggression to another animal that did not originally elicit the aggressive response. The harassed cat may want to attack the feline "bully" but, being afraid to do so, directs its attack to a smaller, younger, or more vulnerable cat in the house. One of our cats, which becomes irritated when forced to get off the kitchen counter (and would not think of attacking us) often walks over to one of the dogs, jumps on his neck, and begins biting him. Fortunately, the Dalmatian thinks this is a great game, and a fun wrestling match ensues.

Unpredictable Environments

Cats in multi-cat households may be vulnerable to frequent conflicts with other cats, creating an unpredictable environment. The cats never know when they may be ambushed, attacked, threatened, or chased. In other species, unpredictable environments have been shown to activate the adrenal glands, causing a stress reaction.

Environments may be unpredictable for other reasons. Attempting to punish a cat after the fact for misbehavior is a common example. Cats, and other animals, associate punishment only with what they are doing at the time the punishment occurs. If taken over to a soiled area on the floor and verbally scolded or hit, the cat does not understand that this aversive treatment is supposed to be connected to the act of eliminating there minutes or hours before. From the cat's point of view, the scolding was associated with whatever it was doing when it was so abruptly picked up. This could be anything from walking across the floor to looking out the window. Thus, the cat can never predict when its owner will come charging out of nowhere because the owner's behavior is not consistent with the cat's behavior. This unpredictable behavior can be a source of stress.

Unfamiliar Environments

Because today's cats share many facets of their owners' lives, it is not uncommon for cats to be taken from their home environment. Cats may go on extended car trips, be flown on airplanes, spend time in hotel rooms, be taken to boarding facilities, accompany their owners during frequent moves, or visit the homes of friends and relatives during vacations and holidays. Cats going to a new home from a shelter, breeder, or previous owner will also be exposed to unfamiliar environments, which have been shown to trigger stress reactions.

The most likely responses under these circumstances are fear-related behaviors, including hiding, defensive aggression, excessive vocalization, excessive elimination, a decrease in eating perhaps to the point of anorexia, "hyper" activity, or freezing, immobile behaviors. Cats that have been well socialized as kittens and exposed in a positive and gentle manner to different environments will probably tolerate changes better than those that have not.

Barren or restricted environments also have been shown to be stressful. Cats that spend much of their time living in cages, kennels, or rooms that do not provide opportunities for them to play, explore, and show a variety of other behaviors may be stressed. Most people would conclude that a cat in a cage that was meowing, pacing, and trying to escape was stressed. Fewer people would reach the same conclusion if a cat was lying quietly, but under these conditions, cats may show behavioral depression and become inactive. Depression also can be a sign of stress.

Separation Distress

Another potential stressor is separation distress. It is normal for all species of social animals to show a distress reaction when separated from other animals to which they have become attached. Vocalizations, attempts to reunite with or gain access to the other animal, and/or depression can be distress reactions. Dogs may show separation distress by becoming destructive, house soiling, or barking excessively when their owners leave for a normal workday. Several certified applied animal behaviorists believe cats are more likely to experience separation distress only when their owners leave for more extended periods, such as for a weekend or a longer vacation. A cat may show a similar reaction after the loss of another family pet to whom it was closely attached. Reported behavioral changes include failure to eat, increased meowing or crying, lack of interest in playing or other daily routines, restlessness, and elimination outside the litter box.

Individual animals react differently to stressors depending on the type of stressor, past experience, and the individual's coping style. Rats, mice, and some farm animals have shown passive and active coping styles in response to stressors. An animal with an active coping style is more likely to develop stereotypes, become aggressive, and be more active in response to stress. A passive coping style is characterized by less activity and increased immobility.

Cautions in Interpretations

The types of stressors and the behavioral responses to them are based on scientific information about many species, including mice, rats, primates, pigs, sheep, and chickens. We've applied this information to similar situations and behaviors in cats because few studies directly linking physiological and behavioral stress responses to specific environmental conditions or events have been conducted with cats.

One study by Dr. Kathy Carlstead demonstrated that irregular feeding and handling schedules, relocation to a new environment, travel in a cat carrier, noise, and lack of petting from care-givers were associated with behavioral changes, with increased concentrations of urinary cortisol, or with both. Her results suggest that consistent routines and predictable environments are very important in minimizing stress responses in cats.

Recommendations

When you are trying to determine if your cat is stressed, keep this discussion in perspective. Many of the behaviors displayed in response to stress are normal behaviors that cats should be expected to show from time to time. Just because your cat doesn't eat for a day, or it urinates outside the litter box, does not necessarily mean the cat is stressed. Experts in stress research all agree that the most accurate way to evaluate stress levels is with a variety of measurements, both behavioral and physiological. Concluding that an animal is stressed based on observations of one behavior change is likely to be wrong.

If your cat shows persistent or significant behavior changes, take the cat to the veterinarian. Illness and disease as stressors producing behavior changes should be considered first. If you know your cat will be subjected to an environmental stressor such as a move, talk to your veterinarian about short-term antianxiety medications or homeopathic remedies to minimize the stress reaction.

We often make assumptions about what is stressful for animals based on what is stressful for us. This tendency may sometimes lead to the wrong conclusion. For example, if asked which of the following would be the most stressful to sheep, what would be your response: being chased by a dog, loaded into a truck, dipped in insecticide, or sheared? The highest cortisol levels were measured in response to shearing, presumably because this involved being separated from the flock. Sheep are highly social, and separation from their group produces strong reactions. We're sure that some of you believed one of the other three events would be the most stressful. This demonstrates that what is stressful will vary among different species of animals.

Finally, remember that stress is not necessarily bad. Stress responses allow animals, including people, to cope with changes in their environment. Change and stress are inevitable. Some scientists believe animals actually benefit from some stress and that a totally stress-free environment may be harmful. The difficulty caring for pets is being able to know when stress is detrimental to an animal's well-being. A definitive answer may not always be available for that complex question.

Perhaps the best guideline is to try to ensure that our family cats are kept in environments that allow them to show us a wide range of their normal behaviors. As an extreme example, cats that spend the majority of their time hiding, lying immobile, fighting, chasing their tails, licking themselves, and chasing or being chased are stressed and are not well off. Cats that occasionally get in skirmishes, refuse to come down from the top of the refrigerator for a day, or get "freaked out" when the family is away for a week at Christmas will probably show signs of stress. At other times, if they are playing, eating, sleeping, exploring, and in general doing activities that cats do, things are probably okay.

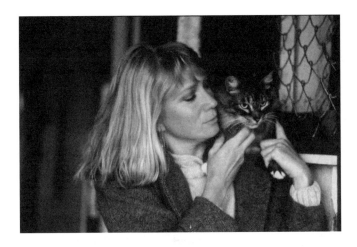

Appendix K

Cat Training Classes: Nine Steps to Celebrate and Protect a Cat's Nine Lives

Step One: Introduction

INTRODUCE YOURSELF, welcome people to the class, and describe what will happen in chronological order (class starts at 6:30 P.M. and runs until 8:00 P.M.):

1. Litter box training.
2. Destructive scratching.
3. Grooming.
4. Preventative healthcare: food, vaccinations, parasite control, dentistry, etc.
5. Sell the project.
   a Make appointment for complimentary veterinary exam and preventive healthcare measures.
   b Pass out free food samples, etc.
   c Detail and sell pet supplies.

Special recognition for this contribution is given to Marty Becker, DVM.

Step Two: Bonding

Bond the client "emotionally" by celebrating the human-animal bond with a graphic touching story.

Ask the client to remember the first cat they ever had. First ask them to remember the cat's name (ask for some names from the audience). Then take them further down this mental road by asking them the breed, color, where it slept, what it ate, when the cat was the happiest, when they were the happiest with the cat, and finally under what circumstances they had to say good-bye.

With great emotion and conviction stress that this human-animal bond is one of the longest-lasting, most powerful, and most significant emotional events in their life. Emphasize that the goal of our having these training classes is to

• Celebrate and protect the human-animal bond.
• We want to be lifelong partners with them in having a happy, healthy pet that is part of the family and that lives life to its fullest potential.

Step Three: Cats Aren't Dogs!

Understand that cats aren't the same as dogs. One is not better than the other, just different.

Difference between dogs and cats? Dogs come when they are called . . .
cats say "take a message" and I'll get back to you!
—Mary Bly

Dogs live to please their owners. Cats live to please themselves.
That's why there are no obedience classes at cat shows!
—Phil Maggitti

Harrison Weir, the Englishman who invented cat shows, believed that cats have a natural, sullen antipathy to being taught, restrained, or made to do anything to which their nature or feelings are averse. Unlike dogs, who in the wild depend on the pack for survival and easily and willingly transfer that interdependence to their human pack, cats are consummate freelancers. Independence suits them just fine. So rather than ask why cats don't come when called, we should ask, instead, why should they?

When should you start training your cat? The best time to start training it is as soon as you have established a rapport with your new feline friend. As soon as your cat has identified you as the source of food and lavish attention, you should begin teaching it to respond to the name you have chosen for it.

Step Four: Litter Training

A sobering fact? The number one reason for convenience euthanasia in cats is for litter box related problems (70–80 percent). Therefore, it is critical that we do everything we can to prevent litter-related problems.

Litter maintenance, litter type, litter box placement, and the number of boxes in the household are some of the most important components in cat ownership.

Many types of litter material are on the market. These include plain clay, plain clay with added odor control substances, scoopable/clumping type, those that can be flushed down the toilet, and pelleted newspaper. The choice of material is up to the cat owner, but certain factors should be considered.

The first is the individual cat. One should take into account that cats can have preferences for litter materials. Some cats are sensitive to odor and do not like scented litters. Therefore, an unscented one would be best. Some cats are more particular about texture and prefer one of the scoopable or clumping brands. Other cats may prefer unusual products like cedar chips, play sand, or even dirt.

It may take a little trial-and-error, but if your cat is comfortable with one kind of litter, stick with that brand and leave the litter pan in the same place. Cats are creatures of habit, and switching litters may result in accidents.

There are three main times when your cat will have the urge to eliminate:

• After eating.
• After waking up.
• After playing.

When your new cat is getting used to its surroundings, place him gently in the litter pan after any of the above to help reinforce his natural instincts. If the cat eliminates, praise it gently but with enthusiasm and love.

Here are the four main reasons a cat won't use the litter box and will have accidents:

1. *Improper cleaning and maintenance.* Cats are clean animals and are sensitive to odor. The best way to control odor is through thorough and frequent cleaning. Therefore, it is important that an owner have a regular pattern of litter maintenance. Although most owners only change the litter material every seven days, for many cats this is not often enough. As a basic rule, the fecal matter should be scooped out daily and the litter changed every four to seven days. When cleaning the pan, it is best to use a mild dish soap (avoid ammonia based cleaners or other strong cleaners that are abhorrent to some cats) or just put the pan outside in the sunlight for 30 minutes to an hour on a regular basis.

2. *The cat is not spayed or neutered.* Unneutered male cats have a strong natural desire to spray urine and mark territory. Female cats exhibit the same behavior only to a much weaker extent. We highly recommend having your pet spayed or neutered, and it can be done safely as early as eight weeks of age. The sooner the better.

3. *The cat has a medical problem.* When a cat suddenly stops using the litter box, the first step should be to take the cat to the veterinarian to rule out a medical problem. Again, the sooner the better!

4. *Instead of Pandora's box, the litter box can be Pandora's pan.* Another cat is in the house, you've moved the pan (or the area doesn't give adequate privacy, is too close to where she eats, or is too close to where she cat-naps), the cat now has access to an upstairs or basement and doesn't feel like traveling very far to eliminate, you've changed brands or litter, bought a new pan, etc.

What if your cat has inappropriate elimination and you discover it with your foot during your midnight bathroom run? Experts recommend that unless you catch your cat in the act (within three to five seconds of having gone), you must ignore the accident. Punishment after the fact will not affect this behavior and will do further harm. If you do catch your cat in the act, reprimand it verbally with a stern "no" or "bad kitty." Then clean the area with a product that will eliminate the odor, not just mask it.

Rules of Thumb

• Find a litter your cat likes and don't change it.
• Clean fecal material out daily and change litter as needed but at least every four to seven days.
• Get a litter box that fits and suits your cat. For example, a small cat may need a box with small sides, and some cats don't like covered boxes. Have one litter box per cat and one litter box per level in the house.
• Get your cat spayed or neutered and always check with a veterinarian immediately if your cat has urination problems.

Our Recommendations

• Lift-n-Sift Cat Pan, BoodaBox, or Doskocil Covered Box.
• Ultra Clump Litter.
• One-Step Cleaner.

Step Five: Scratching

Cats have a strong desire to scratch. Scratching is an inherited, normal behavior of cats. They do it for four primary reasons:

1. Claw conditioning, such as the removal of the dead outer layer of their claws.
2. Visual territorial marking.
3. Olfactory territorial marking, with scent from glands in their paws.
4. Stretching their front limbs. (Ever watch a cat wake up?)

A cat normally chooses a prominent vertical object to scratch and returns again and again to the same location (a tree, for example). The front claws are extended, gripping the surface, and are withdrawn and extended alternately. This action not only leaves a prominent visual mark but also an olfactory mark from secretions of the sweat glands in the paws. This scratching action also aids in the conditioning of claws by removing old, frayed, and loose layers of claw and exposing the sharp, healthy, new claw underneath (cats also chew the old claw off while grooming themselves). The instinct to scratch begins at about one month after birth. So it is important that rather than try to stop cats from scratching, we

• Find an object for them to scratch that is mutually acceptable (e.g., a scratching post).
• Remove their claws, cover them over with protective caps such as Soft Paws, trim their nails frequently.

An Acceptable Place to Scratch

How can you get a cat to use a scratching post? The following rules of thumb will help:

- Because cats frequently scratch and stretch after waking, put the post close to the cat's sleeping area.
- Some cats prefer free standing sleeping perches and climbing areas, whereas others like a post that is hung on furniture or on a door. Whatever your choice, cats prefer a material that is loosely woven so that their claws can hook into the fabric and tear it using long longitudinal strokes. Often carpet is too durable and won't tear; the cat's claws catch, and the cat refuses to use it. Many experts recommend securely fastening upholstery over the carpet. That way as the cat rips through the upholstery into the carpet, the carpet begins to take on the cat's foot pad odor while the cat can still shred the replaceable upholstery. Some other good materials for scratching have sisal, cardboard, wood, or wood composite surfaces. Please note, unless the scratching post is completely destroyed, *don't* replace it. In fact most cats prefer a post that is worn, stringy, and easy to rip. Along with surface texture, location, habit, visual appearance, and olfactory marks attract the cat back to the same location.
- If the cat is reluctant to use the scratching post, positive reinforcement (rewards) should be used to make the post more appealing. Try one or more of the following:
  - Once the cat awakens, use food or a toy as a lure to get the cat to approach the post. Hold the lure part way up the post and wait until the cat stretches or scratches before giving it the reward.
  - If the post has ledges or platforms, food, toys, or catnip can be placed on the ledges or hung from the post. Some experts recommend spraying the post with spray catnip.
  - Rubbing the cat's paws gently on the post helps provide visual and olfactory cues that may attract the cat back for future scratching.
  - If the cat can't be closely supervised, it should be left with its scratching post in a designated kitten-proof area where unwanted damage cannot occur. This area should contain the cat's bedding, food, water, litter pan, and toys (for some cats this may be a room, an entire floor of the house, or maybe only a large cage).

Discouraging Inappropriate Scratching

What if the cat scratches what it's not supposed to, like your favorite couch? Try one or more of the following:

- *Modify the cat's environment.* This is the first step in the correction of problem household scratching. You can allow the cat more access to the outdoors. Or you can move the damaged furniture and replace it with an appropriate scratching surface, thereby maintaining the location habit (the new scratching post should have the same surface as the old scratching surface and be at the same

level; for example, if the cat liked to scratch the fabric on top of the chair, don't replace it with a wooden scratching post at ground level).
- *Behavior modification: Rewards.* Use catnip, toys, treats, or food rewards to attract the cat to use the new, acceptable scratching post.
- *Behavior modification: Punishment.* The principles of effective punishment require
  - That the cat be caught in the act,
  - That the punishment be aversive enough to deter the cat from returning to the spot, and
  - That the cat associate the punishment with the act of scratching, not with the presence of the owner.

Declawing or Covering the Claws

Declawing is a highly controversial issue. Critics claim declawing can trigger chronic physical ailments such as cystitis, asthma, and skin disorders and cause gradual weakening of the muscles of the forelimb, shoulders, and back. They also claim that hunting, balance, fighting, climbing, and feline social relationships are affected adversely by declawing and that every cat can and should be trained to use a scratching post.

However, if an owner is unwilling or unable to prevent or correct problem scratching using the behavioral modification techniques discussed above, declawing may prove to be an acceptable alternative. Declawing also is an effective way to eliminate household clawing during running, jumping, climbing, and playing. To date, all of the negative or critical comments and statements about declawing have been based on hearsay or anecdotal evidence. Since 1985, a number of studies have looked at the effects of declawing on feline behavior and all have found that declawing met the objectives of all cat owners and caused no detrimental behavioral effects. Most scratching problems are greatly reduced or eliminated by declawing. Ninety-six percent of owners of declawed cats are satisfied with declawing, and as many as 70 percent report an improved relationship with their cat. The human-animal bond is strengthened!

Rules of Thumb

- Cats have a strong urge and instinct to scratch. So either train them to scratch on an appropriate surface or have them declawed (or nails covered).
- Because cats like to scratch after awakening, put the scratching post near their bedding. If the cat has access to several levels of the house, have a post on each level.
- Get a scratching post that has a material the cat will like. To encourage the cat to use the post, use rewards or lures.
- If the cat scratches in an unwanted place, use behavior modification.

Our Recommendations

- Have your cat declawed at 8–16 weeks of age at the same time as sterilization.
- If you don't want your cat declawed, cover their claws with protective caps

such as SoftPaws, trim your cat's nails frequently, and use a scratching post (and use rewards and attractants to encourage its use).

Step Six: Cleanliness

Cats spend a lot of time licking themselves in "hard to reach places." Observe one in the act: they seem very determined, but seem to enjoy the process quite a bit! Why do cats groom themselves? To remove dead hair. Usually, it's a good idea to expedite the process by regularly bathing and brushing your cat.

Why Bathe and Brush Your Cat? Some Benefits

- The more hair you remove, the less the cat has to remove. Also there will be less hair all over your house and clothes!
- Regular grooming can help you in training your cat. If the cat is used to being handled and perceives it as a pleasant experience, your other training (litter pan and scratching) will be much easier.

How to Groom Your Cat

- *Start ASAP.* As soon as your cat is settled in, start grooming him for several minutes each day until he is used to being handled.
- *Use a raised and slick surface.* A table or bathroom counter usually works great (don't use the kitchen table or anywhere else the cat is never allowed).
- *Use a slicker brush or comb.* The proper tool depends on the condition of your cat's coat and how often you groom it. Comb or brush in the direction the coat lies and don't apply too much pressure. If the cat is heavily matted or you have a lot of difficulty grooming it, we recommend you seek the services of a professional groomer.
- *If your cat is not declawed, trim its nails frequently.* Hold the cat facing away from you, hold its paw between your thumb and forefingers and push down to extend the claws, cut only the hooked, talon-like part of the claw below the pink blood line.
- *Get your cat used to being bathed.* Although it is not necessary to bathe a cat, most owners do. We recommend the kitchen sink. Put a rubber mat or towel in the bottom and use the spray attachment to bathe your cat (use warm water only). Make sure you rinse your cat thoroughly. To dry your cat, towel dry first. For most short haired cats air drying is fine. For long-haired cats, many people use a hair dryer. For fly-away static hair, rub an antistatic cloth over your cat's coat.

Step Seven: Healthcare

Will Rogers once commented, "I have always felt that the best doctor in the world is the veterinarian. He can't ask his patients what is the matter—he's got to just know."

Veterinarians love animals and have dedicated their lives to protecting them, healing them, and helping them live happy, healthy lives. Although modern veterinary medicine is blessed with sophisticated diagnostic equipment and we are trained to do advanced procedures in orthopedics, cardiology, dermatology, etc., we would much rather prevent problems than try to cure the sick and heal the wounded. Sadly, according to recent American Veterinary Medical Association statistics, 40 percent of owners did not take their cats in for an annual physical examination or for vaccinations! Thus our emphasis and dedication to preventive healthcare.

The Cornerstones of Preventive Healthcare

- *An annual physical exam.* A veterinarian is trained to look past the obvious—to the potential—and can often catch problems early on before they cause unnecessary pain, expense, or worse.
- *Vaccinations.* Kittens get immunity from their mother's milk and are usually protected against disease until they are about eight weeks old. After that, they rely on vaccinations to protect them. To give a simple explanation of a complicated process, vaccinations cause the body to produce protective proteins called antibodies and white blood cells that ingest and remove disease-causing viruses and bacteria.

Use Example of Sand Timer

- *Parasites.* Some parasites such as ticks, fleas, and lice live on the animal, while others such as roundworms, hookworms, and tapeworms live inside the animal. In either case, parasites can cause harm to the animal and to their human friends and should be routinely checked for and removed.
- *Routine dental care.* A cat's teeth should be white and clean, its gums healthy and pink, and its breath, while not sensually pleasing, not repulsive either! Whereas some cat owners are able to regularly brush their pet's teeth, and we recommend you do, most cannot. Therefore we recommend having your cat's teeth professionally cleaned by your veterinarian at least once a year.
- *Knowing when your cat is sick.* Most cat owners are very intuitive, know their cats intimately, and know when they are sick. A few common clues are
  - The cat eliminates outside its pan.
  - The cat refuses to eat.
  - The cat is listless.
  - The cat is not itself.
  - The cat feels "hot" (i.e., has a temperature above 103°F: 101.5°F is considered normal for a cat, just as 98.6°F is for a human).

Although many signs of illness or trauma demand an immediate trip to the veterinarian, if you are unsure, just pick up the phone and call. Better safe than sorry!

Step Eight: Your Cat's Best Interest

It is important, as the spokespersons for your cat's best interests, that we educate you to make informed decisions concerning your cat's health, happiness, and well-being.

Everything your cat needs means much more than treating accidents and illnesses. It means preventing diseases (viral, bacterial, and dental, etc.), preventing or curing behavioral problems (unwanted scratching, improper elimination, etc.), and helping your pet live a happy, healthy life (proper diet, toys, etc).

Our goal is to help "cookbook" the way you get started with your new feline friend so that you don't have to experience many common problems and can "fast forward" to the good times!

We don't consider it a hard sell, we consider it a must sell! Our professional and moral obligation is to recommend everything you need for a happy, healthy pet. Per our professional oath, we not only are kind to animals, but are pledged to prevent pain and suffering as well.

Some of the things we are about to recommend to you are familiar and others are new. To help you understand "the project" and to make your buying decisions more organized and easier, we have prepared a "project sheet" of *everything you need for a happy, healthy cat.*

Go over Cat Project Sheet (e.g., TLC for Cats by Pfizer).

Step Nine: Protect That Bond

We have great reason to celebrate and protect the family/pet bond. We talk to pets like they're humans, we celebrate their birthdays, we let them sleep with us, we carry photos of them in our wallets, and we buy them Christmas gifts. These aren't just pets, they're members of our families!

As we told you earlier, the reason we hold these seminars is because we want to be a partner with your pet and you for a lifetime. And just like your pets, we're always there when you need us!

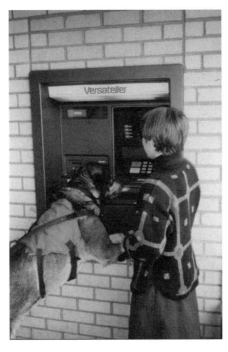

Courtesy of Nancy McKenna
and Delta Society.

Appendix L

Equipment for Behavior Management

T HERE ARE many behavioral products on the market that owners can use to control unruly behaviors and help in training. While a wide variety are listed here, some may be offensive to specific trainers or behaviorists. The equipment list below is not endorsed, nor are all of the methodologies, so the tools and programs must be tailored with your own behavior management consultants.

Humane Training Devices

Promise/Gentle Leader®
 Headcollar

Campbell Pet Co., 800-228-6364
Premier Pet Products, 800-933-5595

Client Handouts

AAHA, 800-883-6301
Lifelearn Diskette: Horwitz and Landsberg,
 800-375-7994

| Child Safety Video | "Dogs, Cats and Kids," Wayne Hunthausen, et al., Amazon.com |
| Clickers | Personalized: LC Advertising, 480-706-1884 Plain, with training kits, bulk: www.Clicker-Company.com, 800-472-5425 |

Direct Interactive Punishment

Barker Breaker (sonic)	Amtek Pet Behavior Products, 11025 Sorrento Valley Court, San Diego, CA, 92121,800-762-7618, 619-597-6681
Direct Stop Repellent (citronella spray)	USA: ABS Inc., 5910-G. Breckenridge Pkwy, Tampa, FL, 33610-4253, 800-627-9447
	CAN: Multivet, P.O. Box 651, St-Hyacinthe, QC, J2S7P5, 800-303-0244, 888-456-2626
Easy Trainer (ultrasonic)	Radio Systems Incorporated, 5008 National Drive, Knoxville, TN, 37914, 800-732-2677, 423-637-8205
K-9 Bark Stopper/Sonic Pet Trainer (sonic)	Innotek, 1000 Fuller Drive, Garrett, Indiana, 46738, 800-826-5527, 219-357-3148
Pet Agree/Dazzer (ultra-sonic)	KII Enterprises, P.O. 306, Camillus, NY 13031, USA: 800-262-3963, 315-468-3596
Ultrasonic Pet Trainer (electronic stimulation)	Radio Systems Incorporated, 5008 National Drive, Knoxville, TN, 37914, 800-732-2677, 423-637-8205

Monitoring Devices

| Tattle Tale (vibration motion sensor) | KII Enterprises, P.O. 306, Camillus, NY 13031, USA: 800-262-3963, 315-468-3596 |

Remote Punishment Collars

ABS Remote Trainer (citronella spray)	USA: ABS, Inc., 5910-G. Breckenridge Pkwy, Tampa, FL, 33610-4253, 800-627-9447; Radio Systems Incorporated, 5008 National Drive, Knoxville, TN, 37914, 800-732-2677, 423-637-8205
	CAN: Sold as Spray Commander by Multivet, P.O. Box 651, St-Hyacinthe, QC, J2S7P5, 800-303-0244, 888-456-2626
Electronic/shock bark collars	Innotek, 1000 Fuller Drive, Garrett, IN, 46738, 800-826-5527, 219-357-3148

Exercise, Play, and Chew Products

Buster Cube	Jorgensen Laboratories Inc., Loveland, CO, 80538, 800-525-5614
Goodie Ship	Space Ball, Planet Pet, P.O. Box 11778, Naples, FL, 800-811-8673
Home Alone Food Ball	Activity Ball, Hightower USA, 4691 Eagle Rock Blvd., Los Angeles, CA, 90041, 800-246-6556, 213-255-1112
Kong Products	Kong Products, 16191-D Table Mountain Parkway, Golden, CO 80403-1641,303-216-2626
Mutt Puck	Mutt Puck, 6260 Reber Place, St. Louis, MO, 63139, 800-274-MUTT, 314-781-MUTT
Nylabone Products	TFH Publications, 1 TFH Plaza, 3rd and Union Ave, Neptune, NJ 07753, 732-988-8400
Pavlov's Cat (cat scratch feeder)	Del-West Enterprises, 1015 Summerwood Court, San Diego, CA 92131, 619-689-9999
Tennis Bone	Happy Dog Toys, P.O. Box 5424, Phoenix, AZ, 85010, 602-585-3511

Booby Traps (Environmental Punishment Devices)

ABS, Indoor and Outdoor Pet Containment Systems (citronella spray)	USA: ABS, Inc. 5910-G. Breckenridge Pkwy, Tampa, FL, 33610-4253, 800-627-9447; Radio Systems Incorporated 5008 National Drive, Knoxville, TN, 37914, 800-732-2677, 423-637-8205
	CAN: Sold as Spray Barrier (indoor citronella spray containment system) and Virtual Fence (outdoor citronella spray system) by Multivet, P.O. Box 651, St-Hyacinthe, QC, J2S7P5, 800-303-0244, 888-456-2626
Innotek, Indoor and Outdoor Pet Containment Systems (electronic stimulation)	Innotek, 1000 Fuller Drive, Garrett, IN, 46738, 800-826-5527, 219-357-3148
Invisible Fencing, Indoor and Outdoor Pet Containment Systems (electronic stimulation)	USA: Invisible Fence Co., 355 Phoenixville Pike, Malvern, PA, 19355, 610-651-0999
	CAN: Trans Canada Pet Boundaries, 905-983-3647
Pet Mat	Radio Systems Incorporated, 5008 National Drive, Knoxville, TN, 37914, 800-732-2677, 423-637-8205

Radio Systems Incorporated, Indoor and Outdoor Pet Containment Systems (electronic stimulation)

Radio Systems Incorporated, 5008 National Drive, Knoxville, TN, 37914, 800-732-2677, 423-637-8205
Veterinary Distribution: DermaPet, 8909 Iveleigh Ct., Potomac, MD, 20854, 800-755-4738

Scat Mat (electronic stimulation mat)

Contech Electronics, P.O. Box 115, Saanichton, BC, V8M 2C3, Canada, 800-767-8658, 604-652-0755

ScareCrow (motion activated sprinkler)

Contech Electronics, P.O. Box 115, Saanichton, BC, V8M 2C3, Canada, 800-767-8658, 604-652-0755

Scraminal/Critter Gitter

Amtek Pet Behavior Products, 11025 Sorrento Valley Ct., San Diego, CA 92121, 800-762-7618, 619-5977-6681

Smart Bowl

Aqcon Inc., 340 Kingswood Road, Toronto, Ontario, M4E 3N9, 416-691-0558, 800-891-2695

Snappy Trainer

Interplanetary Incorporated, 12441 West 49th St., Suite 8, Wheatridge, CO, 80033, 888-477-4738, 303-940-3228

SofaSaver

Abbey Enterprises, 235 West 1st Street, Bayonne, NJ 07002, 201-823-3690

Ultrasonic Pest Deterrent

Radio Systems Incorporated, 5008 National Drive, Knoxville, TN, 37914, 800-732-2677, 423-637-8205

Bark Deterrents

A.B.S. (citronella spray collar)

USA: ABS Inc., 5910-G. Breckenridge Pkwy, Tampa, FL, 33610-4253, 800-627-9447
CAN: Sold as Aboistop (citronella spray collar) by Multivet, P.O Box 651, St-Hyacinthe, QC, J2S7P5, 800-303-0244, 888-456-2626

K-9 Bark Stopper (audible bark activated)

Innotek, 1000 Fuller Drive, Garrett, IN, 46738, 800-826-5527, 219-357-3148

Electronic stimulation bark collars

Radio Systems Incorporated, 5008 National Drive, Knoxville, TN, 37914, 800-732-2677, 423-637-8205
Veterinary Distribution: DermaPet, 8909 Iveleigh Ct., Potomac, MD, 20854, 800-755-4738

Silencer Bark Activated Collar
  (ultrasonic bark activated collar)

Super Barker Breaker
  (audible bark activated)

Radio Systems Incorporated, 5008 National Drive, Knoxville, TN, 37914, 800-732-2677, 423-637-8205

Amtek Pet Behavior Products, 11025 Sorrento Valley Ct., San Diego, CA 92121, 800-762-7618, 619-5977-6681

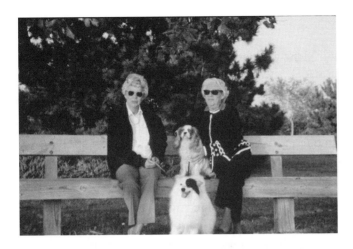

Appendix M

Pet Health Insurance: An Alternative to Economic Euthanasia

What Is It?

ETHICAL PET insurance is a "risk sharing" property insurance, the same as car or home insurance, and that is exactly how it is registered in every state. Ethical pet insurance does *not* require the practice to subscribe or offer a discount; in fact, it is illegal for *anyone* to ask a veterinary practice to sell insurance. To sell insurance, a state license is required. The insurance is owned by the pet owner, even when it is offered as an employee benefit, so it can be used with *any* legally licensed veterinarian. The clients pay the veterinary practice, get an invoice when they pay the bill, and submit the invoice for reimbursement; with the oldest company, wellness care is usually processed and a reimbursement check is mailed in less than a week, and catastrophic care is usually reimbursed within two weeks.

Is It Here to Stay?

The oldest company, Veterinary Pet Insurance (VPI), has over 18 years as a veterinary-specific pet insurance company. They are growing in a logarithmic fashion since they introduced the wellness programs. Their reimbursement tables are based on actual veterinary profession fees and offer a substantial savings to clients whenever an unexpected medical or surgical event occurs. For the increasing number of seniors, often living on a fixed income, in our pet-owning population, insurance allows a very effective allocation of discretionary income on a monthly, quarterly, or annual premium basis.

Why Should We Promote It?

When pet insurance only offered catastrophic coverage, it was an alternative to euthanasia, but with the wellness now offered, it makes economic sense for all people who perceive their pet as a companion and a family member. The VPI wellness reimbursement is more than double the wellness premiums (vendor subsidies do help this), and in fact, approximately covers the total cost of both portions of the insurance premiums. The VPI wellness premium (less than $100) allows the client to send in wellness care invoices, from the licensed veterinarian of their choice, that can result in reimbursement of over $200. Pet owners with pet insurance access veterinary healthcare services almost 50 percent more often than non–insurance owners and spend about 56 percent more per pet. But to me, it has *always* been a caring alternative to euthanasia caused by low available family funds at a crisis time.

How Can We Sell It?

As stated above, a practice should not try to "sell" insurance in any form; that requires a state license. A "caring veterinary provider" discusses with clients the availability, and maybe even the value, of reputable pet insurance and provides the phone numbers of at least two reputable firms (e.g., Veterinary Pet Insurance or Pets*Health*), so the clients can explore at their leisure and make their own decision to purchase or not.

When Their Worry Appears to Be the Cost

♪♪♪ How Much Is That Doggy In The Window ♪♪♪

The tail will keep wagging if we can give clients an economical way to spend their small amount of discretionary income on their pets. When clients call, they do not want to hear the laborious explanation of an untrained receptionist of why the practice's prices are so high; good pet owners want the best value for the best price. So please, answer their question directly, using ideas from the following dialogues:

Q: How much is a dentistry?
A: Do you have pet medical health insurance?
Q: No, why?
A: Because if you did, our adolescent dental would be less than $50 after reimbursement!

Q: How much are the annual vaccinations?

A: Do you have pet medical health insurance?

Q: No, why?

A: Because if you did, our annual booster series, with a doctor's consultation, would be less than $20 after reimbursement!

Q: I saw the Purnia Silver Pet ad about annual blood testing; what is the cost?

A: Do you have pet medical health insurance?

Q: No, why?

A: Because if you did, our full blood chemistry would be less than $20 after reimbursement!

Supplemental and Optional Statements

Since you are worried about cost, let me send you a pet insurance brochure, and if it looks right for you, please call the company. It is not practice exclusive, so if you need to use an emergency practice, or we need to refer your pet to a specialist, the insurance is still in effect.

Since you want the best price, the wellness care portion of this policy provides over $2 of reimbursement for every dollar of premiums . . . two dollars back for every one spent is the best deal on the street today! They also have monthly payment plans.

Pet insurance premiums are age dependent, so for $10 to $15 a month, you can receive coverage for sickness, injury, and wellness care, and with over $215 dollars of wellness care reimbursement available a year, even if your pet does not get sick or injured, you can receive more in reimbursements than you paid in premiums.

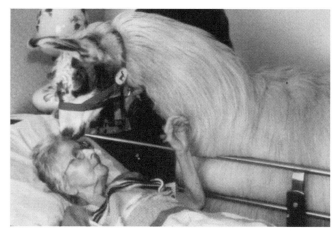

Courtesy of
Delta Society

Appendix N

Help! My Grieving Client Needs Help . . .

A S A veterinarian, I know it is the client who has lost a pet and wants our professional counsel that stretches our abilities to the limit; we haven't been trained to treat a broken heart. When the Delta Society was formed in 1981, I was one of the first in line; I knew I needed the knowledge they networked concerning the human–companion animal bond. I have been at most of the annual meetings of the Delta Society; their meetings have always given me a recharge that rejuvenates the soul. I am also a charter member of the new American Association of Human–Animal Bond Veterinarians, and I watch their e-mail board for activity, which is not too frequent. But what is a practice to do?

How Important Is the Pet?

Before we can adequately counsel grieving clients, we need to be aware of the value of companion animals to those who are suffering loss. We also need to be aware of the stages of grief they will experience in coming to terms with their loss. To this end, the results of the following survey help acquaint us with perceptions of a general population group in comparison with a retired group, a growing segment of pet owners. The value of using companion animals in hospice facilities is presented, as well as the potential support a pet can offer in the grief process. For practical application of this information, there is a section on resource networking related to the grieving process and a section on implementing a grief counseling program in your community at the end of this appendix.

The Value of Pets

The survey used in the introduction of this text allowed us to evaluate 156 retired (over 50 years of age) military families, identify their specific values toward their pets, and compare them to the survey population in total (n=961). In comparing results for the older retired family to those for the total populations, some trends become evident. It was reported that 24.5% usually celebrate their pet's birthday (about 10% less than for the general population surveyed), and when asked about display of their pet's picture, 58% displayed pictures in their homes. These rates reflect more pictures but less birthday celebration than in the total population surveyed, an indication of increased pet importance with less desire to "count the days." A subjective review of the names that the elderly respondents gave their pets, as indicated in the survey, showed that 48% of the pets had "people-type" names, 31% had been named after "things or physical traits," and 21% were given "animal-type" names. When these responses were compared to those of the total population, which reported that 23.4% of pets were named after physical characteristics, 11.7% after TV show/movie/cartoon/book characters, 9% after a person, and 7.7% after a previous pet, the "belonging" status of the pet became far more evident. This was reinforced when the elderly were asked about reasons for selecting their companion animals; they rated the reasons, in order or priority, as follows: pleasure (36%), companionship (35%), and protection (10%).

Table N.1. Characteristics displayed by pets in total and elderly survey populations

Total Population (N=961)		Elderly Population (N=156)
Great Display of Trait	Characteristic	Great Display of Trait
89.3%	Greets you upon coming home	90.6%
76.9%	Pet understands when you talk to him/her	84.4%
72.9%	Communicates to you	78.1%
59.6%	Demands attention	55.4%
59.2%	Understands/is sensitive to your moods	62.9%
49.7%	Stays close when you're anxious or upset	49.5%
44.9%	Sleeps with family member	32.3%
22.5%	Mimics your emotions	20.7%
11.8%	Hides or withdraws when you are anxious or upset	5.1%
10.5%	Expresses feelings that you cannot/do not	16.1%
3.8%	Develops illness when family tension is high	5.1%

Many traits or attributes are credited to the companion animal during daily conversations, so the survey asked specifically what special characteristics the pet displayed with the family. The responses were placed on a line scale from "great" through "some" to "none," with the results as shown in Table N.1.

Table N.2. Importance of pet to total and elderly survey populations in specific situations

Situation	Total Population		Elderly Population	
	Great	None	Great	None
At all times	75.4%	1.7%	79.6%	0.0%
Temporary absence of spouse	73.1%	6.7%	70.6%	5.9%
Free time/relaxation	71.5%	2.8%	78.7%	0.0%
Childhood period	69.6%	9.7%	59.0%	19.7%
Sad, lonely, depressed	68.4%	5.1%	72.3%	4.0%
Marriage without children	58.6%	25.5%	58.5%	24.5%
Temporary absences of children	53.2%	17.5%	51.6%	18.8%
During illness/after death of other	52.0%	13.2%	60.0%	8.2%
During crisis/separation/divorce	50.3%	16.3%	53.3%	18.3%
During moves or relocations	48.2%	17.5%	44.1%	20.3%
Teenage period	44.4%	16.1%	47.5%	18.6%
Unemployment	35.6%	31.4%	34.0%	37.7%

When asked directly to evaluate how important their pet was to their life, 50% reported "extremely important," 34% "very important," 14% "important," and 1.9% moderate to no importance. To better evaluate the importance of the companion animal, respondents were asked to rate the importance of their pet to them, in specific situations, on a line scale from "great" to "some" to "none," with the results as shown in Table N.2.

It was interesting to note that while the intensity of feelings concerning the importance of the companion animal was often more polarized in the elderly than in the population in general, the death of the animal was over 20% less significant to the elderly (73.1% vs. 94.4% important to extreme loss) than to the population in general. This is thought to be due to the greater acceptance of the death process by the elderly.

Besides questions concerning the importance of the pet to specific situations, other questions were posed to evaluate the respondents' anthropomorphic tendencies. When asked how the companion animal fit into the family group, 71.9% stated that the pet had full family member status, 23.9% had friend status, and 3.2% of the pets were considered possessions/owned property. While these responses indicated a greater value to the elderly retired population, 99% of the families surveyed felt children should have pets. Later in the survey, the question was rephrased, and the respondents were asked if pets were afforded "people" status in the family. A line scale was used, and the respondents were asked to rate the status from "always" through "usually" and "sometimes" to "never." The survey indicated 78.4% of the elderly felt their pet was usually to always afforded "people" status, while only 2.6% stated they never gave their pet "people" status; this rate was about 10% higher than for the total surveyed population.

Companion Animals in Hospice Facilities

The hospice approach offers one alternative in the production and delivery of medical services to the terminally ill, regardless of age. Attention is focused on palliative rather than curative care, offering death with dignity. In addition, several elements of care usually not found in the acute care system are part of the hospice: treatment of family and patient as one unit, continuum of care, symptom management and pain control, use of the interdisciplinary team, utilization of therapy extenders or facilitators, and bereavement counseling. Many of these benefits, such as the effects of using companion animals, are difficult to measure. While the literature is full of articles about the role of animals with the elderly or with children, death is seldom mentioned.

Utilization of companion animals to reduce feelings of loneliness, depression, or boredom has been well documented in recent literature. The elderly with companion animals perceive less loneliness and less emotional isolation; they also have something to care for, to keep them busy, to watch in idle times, and/or to provide a stimulus for exercise. Individuals in elder care facilities have also exhibited dramatic improvements in their ability to interact and communicate with other residents and staff. These behavioral effects, whether subjectively or objectively proven, have resulted in a decreased staff workload, as well as an improved cost-benefit ratio. This animal-facilitated communication benefit could assist hospice teams at any point in the Kubler-Ross loss phenomenon shown below. (See Table N.3 for a listing of potential roles for companion animals in this grief/loss process.) Furthermore, the importance of the companion animal in life review, or reminiscence, cannot be understated in the hospice program; the animal provides a sense of security, as well as a dependence that often anchors the hospice patient to the realities of life.

Kubler-Ross Loss Phenomenon
in Death/Dying Bereavement
(Stress Mediated)

DENIAL
ANGER
GUILT
DEPRESSION
ACCEPTANCE

The Grief Process

Grief is a process, not a single feeling. It is a process of letting go within the life process. It is important for us as veterinarians to understand the positive role companion animals can play during a period of loss (see Table N.3, below). It is also important for us to be aware of the stages of grief experienced during the loss. These stages are shown in Table N.4.

Table N.3. Potential roles of animals in the grief process

Companionship
Nonjudgmental love
Security/safety
Neutral communication point
Stress reduction
Triangulation (third party role)
Reality anchor during reminiscence
Potential distractions (e.g., exercise)
Intangible distractions (e.g., mood)
Mandatory distractions (e.g., feeding care)
Stability of environment

Networking for Resources

As a veterinarian you can network for grief counseling resources: You join the Delta Society (Renton, WA, 800-869-6898) and get their resource list for grief counseling. You also join the American Association of Human–Animal Bond Veterinarians (request your application on NOAH or VIN). You then buy the books, get the journals, and become astute at the "first aid" level of counseling— learn to listen and ask questions that allow clients to discover the solution for themselves. But what of the practice team?

The American Animal Hospital Association (1-800-252-2242) released a three-tape VCR series, Pet Loss and Bereavement. The first 45-minute tape discusses pet loss and the grief process; the second reflects on methods that the practice team can use to counsel and console clients. Each of these tapes comes with a unique workbook that is veterinary practice specific; they allow the practice to tailor its approach to fit the practice philosophy. The third tape in the series is designed to be sent home with the client and has a brochure for the client to review. It is a great aid during those anticipatory grief times, when you first discover the cancer, or when the family must relocate and leave the pet behind, or when the congestive heart failure first becomes symptomatic. These tapes are a must for any practice that wants a team approach to client bereavement and wants to help the client decide to return to the practice. The "new" AAHA study replicated (with an 80 percent smaller sample) the same family values published

Table N.4. The stages of grief and the key players at each stage

	Anticipatory Grief Stage	Crisis Grief Stage	Crucible Grief Stage	Reconstruction Grief Stage
Event	Death is expected	Death occurs	After the funeral	Return to self senses
Emotions	Denial with hope Hope with long range spiritual plan Anger and/or guilt Withdrawal and social death as rehearsal Overcompensations become smothering	Shock Numbness Disorientation Disbelief	Pain and fear Blame and anger Guilt Reminiscence Need to deal with emotional realities Develop new roles for family members	Orientation to present New interests Self-growth *Getting stuck signs:* Two weeks of insomnia Increased weight loss Increased booze Increased destructive behavior
Key players	Family Ministry	Healthcare provider Funeral director	Social counselors Ministry Significant others	The person him/herself

in the *Pet Connection,* the 1983 Delta Society proceedings text (Catanzaro 1984). *Universal Kinship: The Bond between All Living Things* (Latham Foundation) shares additional viewpoints and tools from multiple authors about the human-animal bond. In the chapter on grief, the stages of grief, from anticipatory to crisis to crucible to reconstructive, are explained; also included are certain practice actions which should be considered (see Table N.5).

In most family pet loss situations, grief is severe. The pet was a member of the family and has been lost. The pain felt is the price paid for the love shared; but that doesn't reduce the pain. In most people, the grief process is a series of natural reactions (see Table N.4), as explained by Kubler-Ross in her landmark textbook, *On Death and Dying.* These are seen in each of the client stages shown in Table N.5. But in some cases, certain people "get stuck" in one of the stages of grief (see Table N.4); this is beyond our "first aid" counseling capabilities. The practice team generally cannot be effective at this time of crisis; the client isn't listening to anyone. What can you do, and where can a practice go for help?

In every community there are psychologists, social workers, and other professionals who are trained to communicate with people who are stuck in some phase of grief. How do you find these skilled professionals that are needed by your clients?

Table N.5. Stages of grief for loss of pet

Client Stage	Practice's Response
Normal examination needed	Patient advocacy—caring team becomes aware of potential loss—anticipatory grief
Pet enters crisis stage	Offers counsel—provides VCR—helps client accept the healthcare situation —empathy—caring
Pet is lost	Empathy—quiet presence—caring—disposition assistance
Family tries to adapt	Sympathy card—referral
Good memories outweigh pain	Foundation letter—phone call

Selling the Concept Locally

Many veterinary schools have developed a fully coordinated grief counseling program at the veterinary teaching hospital; some VMAs have programs that link veterinarians with the grief counseling professionals in the community [e.g., Denver Area Veterinary Medical Society (DAVMS)]. This allows both professional teams to use the resources of the other. The Pet Loss cohort groups start monthly, at an economical cost for the client who has lost his/her pet. The group meets for eight weekly sessions and then it disbands. If any individual still has a critical need, the group facilitator has the resources available to refer the client to individual sessions. But how do you start such an interprofessional team, in your own community?

To make it work, regardless of the community size, talk to your colleagues and use your local veterinary medical association; at a meeting, show an extract from the AAHA VCR tape(s) and share the excitement of the DAVMS program. Armed with the Delta Society resource list and the AAHA pet loss tapes, seek out a few local family counselors and sell your concept. These professionals understand the dynamics of family loss and have a professional group that can also network a support system; the profit motive can be addressed at this time to make the excitement really happen. Use the concepts of the DAVMS success story and offer to work to develop the same interprofessional system. Your local veterinary association makes the economies of scale workable and keeps it cost effective for all concerned. A joint meeting should be scheduled with key players from each group to outline the mechanics of the referral system. The DAVMS has developed a client brochure that is in most veterinary reception areas in the greater Denver metroplex; often the program sells itself.

There are many facets to bereavement, and many start in the stress of daily life. Developing a bereavement counseling capability within a veterinary practice will generally extend the same team skills to daily activities, such as the hit-by-car crisis or the pampered poodle's panicked owner. It doesn't matter. The people skills we learn to use in bereavement situations are identical to those we must use in stress situations; this includes the Saturday morning practice rush. You owe it to your team to develop these skills; it will enhance client relations as well as staff relationships.

References

Catanzaro, T.E. 1984. A Study of the Human/Companion Animal Bond in Mobile Military Families in the United States. In *The Pet Connection: Its Influence on Our Health and Quality of Life,* ed. R.K. Anderson, B.L. Hart, and L.A. Hart. Minneapolis: Center to Study Human-Animal Relationships and Environments (CENSHARE), University of Minnesota.

Kubler-Ross, E. 1997. (Reprint edition.) *On Death and Dying.* Collier Books.

Latham Foundation. 1992. *Universal Kinship: The Bond Between All Living Things.* R&E Publishers.

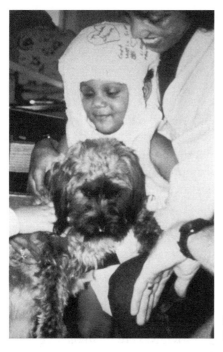

Courtesy of T. Sam Houston
Hospital and Delta Society.

Appendix O

What Do I Tell the Children?

Seneca said it, animals do it. "Begin at once to live, and count each separate day as a separate life." *Caring staff help clients understand this and celebrate the life that was.*

A S a veterinarian, the hardest question at the examination table doesn't deal with a patient, it deals with the patient's family. The clients, their children, and others who depend on the animal's nonjudgmental love undergo severe stress when the patient becomes a critical healthcare case. The grief associated with a terminal illness or death causes that toughest of questions: *"What do I tell the children?"*

The Academic Answer

If we read the cursory literature, we are told to be truthful. The concept is solid and the need critical, but those cursory pamphlets don't tell us how to deliver this truth. A truth delivered without sensitivity is a way to lose clients. A caring concern that contains the truth helps us retain our clients.

What is the truth? Fluffy was "put to sleep" by the veterinarian is the worst form of truth. Many children will then fear sleep, blame the veterinarian, or in some cases, expect the pet to return when they reawaken. Why do we continue to support this euphemism?

"The veterinarian thought it was best to put Fluffy out of her misery." Again, here is a truth that conjures up a fear of becoming hurt in children, a fear of telling Mom that the stomach pains are causing them misery. The shifting to why answers will generally cause referral of responsibility, an avoidance of personal participation in the decision process. Children need to know the truth, but at their level of understanding.

The Caring Response

Don't "give" the children the truth; instead, answer each question honestly. A child's ability to understand is dependent upon both personal experience and knowledge development. The age groupings provided herein are only general, since each child is on a continuum of development that is completely dependent upon his/her specific life experiences.

Preschool

Preschoolers usually do not comprehend the idea of absence of life. Often television analogies confuse the concepts we offer. The children make very literal interpretations of adult euphemisms and very easily accept self-blame, which cannot be explained away. Preschool children need to be told in terms that relate to experiences they understand, but do not give them more information than they request. Repetition of questions will be common as children struggle to understand this new concept of death. Parents, relatives, and siblings need to be consistent in answering questions in order to minimize misconceptions.

Early School Age

Children at this age understand death is final, can identify specific external causes, believe death is a gradual process, (often happening only to others), and personify death as a spirit role like a ghost or bogeyman. They may believe they can cause death by wishes or ill feelings, show increased interest in the permanence of death, and role play in death rituals. They may also misunderstand euphemisms, although they realize the assumed meanings contradict the evidence. Early school-aged children will understand a pet is dead, but they may need concrete evidence of the death. Encourage five- to nine-year-olds to ask questions about anything they do not understand, but answer at their level of knowledge and experience. Parents should support exploration and play related to death and keep teachers informed of potential grief reactions so they can be consistent and caring.

Older School-aged Children (10-plus Years)

This is the age where abstract thinking begins; these older school-aged children use ideas, theories, and logical relationships to explain their experiences. They understand that death will happen to all living things, eventually, that it may be immediate rather than gradual, and that it can occur suddenly and without warning. The children begin to accept the natural cessation of life functions as the cause of death and are capable of understanding religious or philosophical concepts, such as heaven or rituals. Older school-aged children have a good understanding of death and should be encouraged not only to ask questions, but also to express their thoughts and feelings. Children at 10 years and older are capable of participating in decisions about euthanasia or disposal of the body and should be consulted before and after the euthanasia and/or final disposition.

Support Systems

There are many ways to support the family and children at the time of the loss of a loved one. *Kids Grieve Too!* by V.S. Lombardo and E.F. Lombardo (1986, Charles C. Thomas, Springfield, Illinois) is one of the most recent references, and *Talking with Young Children About Death* by F. Rogers and H.B. Sharapan (1979, Family Communications of Pittsburg) is one of the cornerstone references. Texts that can help parents are provided in a supplemental bibliography, and the ones that fit your practice style must fit the needs of your clients. To provide choices appropriate for different practice needs, a large selection is provided. The fact that *The Tenth Good Thing About Barney* works well for me doesn't mean it will fit well for you or for the client who has only hunting dogs.

Start reading now, and use the grief library as you would the chemotherapeutics on your pharmacy shelf. Pick the one that best intercedes in the process to help the recovery of the client.

Books to Help Children Cope with the Death of a Pet

The following books depict children as they deal with the death of a pet. Adults may wish to review books before sharing them with children, in order to find those which are most suited to individual situations.

Abbott, S. 1972. *The Old Dog.* New York: Coward. After his dog dies, Ben realizes there is a difference between death and sleeping. Ben's grieving time is cut short when his father brings home a new puppy. Ages 4–8.

Armstrong, W.H. 1969. *Sounder.* New York: Harper. After the deaths of his father and the family dog, a boy's memories of both become valuable tools in dealing with future experiences. Ages 10–14.

Brown, M.W. 1958. *The Dead Bird.* Reading, MA: Addison-Wesley. This classic book addresses death with simplicity. A group of children find a dead bird and carry out an elaborate funeral. Ages 4–8.

Carrick, C. 1976. *The Accident.* New York: Seabury. A boy deals with anger and sorrow after his dog is killed by a truck. Ages 5–8.

Cate, D. 1976. *Never Is a Long, Long Time.* New York: Thomas Nelson. Billy's father eventually agrees to get him a new puppy after the death of his old dog. Ages 9–11.

Fairless, C. 1980. *Hambone.* Plattsburg, NY: Tundra. Jeremy copes with the death of his pet pig by planting a memorial tomato seedling in Hambone's honor. Ages 8–11.

Gackenbach, D. 1975. *Do You Love Me?* New York: Seabury. The accidental death of a hummingbird helps Walter see that not all animals want to be pets. Ages 5–9.

Graeber, C.T. 1982. *Mustard.* New York: Macmillan. Alex's parents are supportive and honest as they help him cope with the illness and death of his cat, Mustard. Ages 4–10.

Hall, L. 1976. *Flowers of Anger.* New York: Follett. A girl's anger and sorrow after her horse is killed distance her from her best friend. Ages 10–12.

Hegwood, M. 1975. *My Friend Fish.* New York: Holt, Rinehart and Winston. A young boy encounters death for the first time when his pet fish dies. Ages 6–9.

Hurd, E.T. 1980. *The Black Dog Who Went Into The Woods.* New York: Harper and Row. A young boy, along with the rest of his family, copes with feelings of loss after Black Dog dies. Ages 5–7.

Little, M.E. 1979. *Old Cat and the Kitten.* New York: Atheneum. Joel's strong sense of responsibility and loyalty are shown as he must choose between euthanasia and abandonment for his cat. Ages 8–12.

Rawlings, M.K. (1938). *The Yearling.* New York: Scribner. Jody must kill his beloved pet fawn when it begins to destroy the family's crops. Ages 12+.

Rogers, Fred 1988. *When a Pet Dies.* New York: G.P. Putnam's Sons. First experiences picture book from Mister Rogers' Neighborhood series, exploring the feelings of frustration, sadness, and loneliness that a youngster may feel when a pet dies. Ages 4–9. (Available from AAHA, PO Box 150889, Denver, CO 80215-0899.)

Simon, S. 1976. *Life and Death in Nature.* New York: McGraw-Hill. Simple experiments that help children explore decomposition, ecology, and the balance of life are described. Ages 6–10.

Stull, E. 1964. *My Turtle Died Today.* New York: Holt. The cycle of life is emphasized, as the death of a pet turtle is followed by the birth of kittens. Ages 3–6.

Thiele, C.M. 1978. *Storm Boy.* New York: Harper and Row. In Australia, a boy raises an orphaned pelican. His fond memories of the bird are great comfort after it is shot by a hunter. Ages 8–11.

Tobias, T. 1978. *Petey.* New York: Putnam. Emily's parents help her cope with the illness and death of her pet gerbil. Ages 6–9.

Viorst, J. 1971. *The Tenth Good Thing about Barney.* New York: Atheneum. A boy is encouraged to remember good things about his cat after it dies. Ages 5–9. (Available from AAHA, PO Box 150899, Denver, CO 80215-0899.)

Wagner. J. 1969. *J.T.* New York: Van Nostrand Reinhold. A young boy feels a sense of being needed as he cares for an injured alley cat. His parents attempt to comfort him after the cat is hit by a car. Ages 8–10.

Wallace, B. 1980. *A Dog Called Kitty.* New York: Holiday House. Kitty has helped Ricky overcome his fear of dogs. After Kitty is killed, Ricky eventually accepts a new puppy. Ages 9–11.

Warburg, S.S. 1969. *Growing Time.* Boston: Houghton Mifflin. Jamie needs time to adjust to his old dog's death and at first rejects the new puppy. Ages 5–9.

Wilhelm, Hans. 1985. *I'll Always Love You.* Belgium: Crown Publishing. The family's story of Elfie, from puppy through life and into death, and the family's feelings. Ages 4–12. (Available from AAHA, PO Box 150899, Denver, CO 80215-0899.)

Winthrop, E. 1975. *A Little Demonstration of Affection.* New York: Harper and Row. A brother and sister are drawn closer together after their dog is shot. Ages 12–16.

White, E.B. 1952. *Charlotte's Web.* New York: Harper. Wilbur the pig is saved from death by the cleverness of his spider friend, Charlotte. Later Charlotte dies, and Wilbur is comforted by friendship with her children. Ages 7+.

Young, J. 1974. *When the Whale Came to My Town.* New York: Knopf. The death of a beached whale is depicted as part of the natural order of things. Ages 6–10.

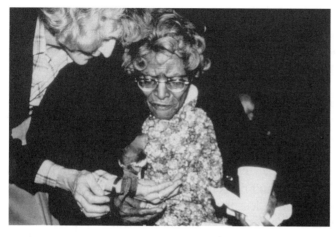

Appendix P

Pet-Mediated Stress Therapy: A Practice Builder

THE PRESCRIPTION, "Take two pets and call me in the morning," may not be far away, since the acceptance of the human-animal bond has become an interdisciplinary fact. With the ever increasing number of successful pet-mediated medical therapies being reported, it is often difficult to remember that this alternative form of treatment is only adjunctive therapy to a skilled healthcare professional. The human-animal bond programs are not a panacea for the healthcare delivery of tomorrow, but they do hold an important role for veterinary healthcare representatives. With the advent of the interdisciplinary healthcare professional team, alternative modalities such as pet facilitated therapy are becoming an acceptable need rather than the luxury of a few.

The Pet Therapist

Animals have been used to reduce feelings of stress, loneliness, depression, or boredom since the late 1800s in Europe, and their use has been well documented in the literature of the Delta Society and related publications (CENSHARE 1984, Fogle 1981, Honori and Beck 1983). The behavioral changes associated with the introduction of animals, whether subjectively or objectively proven, generally result in a reduced staffing requirement. The harmony and tranquility, as well as the increased communications, that accompany an animal facilitated therapy program

183

improve the quality time ratio for each patient and staff member. This leads to a secondary subjective benefit of an improved cost-benefit ratio due to the reduced need for stress therapy, whether chemical or personal. When one looks at the role of the animal in relation to the long-accepted Kubler-Ross loss phenomenon seen during stress or bereavement (denial, anger, guilt, depression, acceptance), the benefits of a "pet therapist" become readily apparent.

The sequence of emotions experienced with a loss cannot be isolated to medical conditions. For example, look at an average teenager. It is final exam time, and our teenager knows the teacher can't flunk him . . . then gets angry when the fact is put out that achieving anything less than 100 percent on the final will result in a failing grade. The teacher is out to get him . . . but then, on the way home, the realization hits that his folks have been pushing the homework in lieu of the phone every night for a full month; guilt sets in quickly. Our teenager gets home, storms through the house muttering about a miserable teacher, heads to his room, and slams the door. The depression and remorse begin to set in and the teenager starts to feel sorry for himself. A noise at the door distracts him; it is the dog scratching to get in to say hello. As the dog enters, the "brightness" of the room improves, the mood changes, and our teenager vents his feelings to the dog. The dog sits and wags the famous happy tail. Acceptance is reached after an in-depth discussion with the dog . . . but it doesn't help at all facing Dad. As the discussion with Dad goes from bad to worse, the dog decides he needs to go out for a walk, and our teenager quickly seizes the opportunity to escape. During the walk, after another discussion with Mr. Dog, our teenager gets to the bargaining stage of resolution (and Dad's temper has cooled a little with the help of Mom back home). When the family gets back together, a compromise is struck, and the dog makes the rounds of a happier family group.

Teenagers generally don't talk to authority figures about their depression or anger. In our younger days, "they" didn't talk to us either. Throughout time, the family pet has had the waiting ear and has provided the nonjudgmental love so critical to youth, and even to adults, although we often don't want to admit it. Talking the crisis through with a pet often creates a new perspective that leads to a resolution of the stress situation. In cases of stuttering children, geriatric patients, cardiac care patients, hospice situations, or depression cases, the pet therapist stands ready to listen and love.

The Hospice Situation

Hospice is a family-oriented healthcare program that provides support to patients with terminal illnesses. The nonjudgmental love of animals can make the difference for a family working through the stress and grief associated with losing a loved one. The animal will interact with the patient as if he/she were a real important person, not a sickly patient. This is a critical factor in any hospice situation. The pet will help the family by being there for warmth and companionship and also will often provide a neutral topic for communication with the patient.

The scientific use of animals in hospice programs could be evaluated from either the perspective of the patient's needs or the needs of the family. Regardless, the key factor in any animal facilitated program is acceptance by all the participants: patient, family, therapists, and veterinary healthcare provider. The veterinary representative and hospice team must interview all the people who will interact with the animal(s), whether it is a new companion animal or an existing family pet. If consensus cannot be reached early, the veterinary healthcare representative must educate the participants about the expected benefits and ensure the hospice team and patient-family group understand the companion animal's role as an adjunctive therapy alternative.

Cost-effective Quality Care

Healthcare costs have risen 700 percent since 1965, with hospital charges now exceeding $150 billion each year. The cost of the average hospital stay soared from $670 to over $3000 between 1970 and 1980. Using animals to reduce the length of stay or the intensity of treatment allows healthcare costs to be maintained rather than escalated in these times of spiraling prices.

The search for alternative treatment modalities to save money has led to the acceptance of animal facilitated therapy programs, hospice programs, and an increase in outpatient procedures. Concurrent with the cost-saving considerations, there has been an awakening to a more realistic attitude toward death and quality of life factors. The companion animal improves the quality of life in virtually every household and becomes very important to households under stress. The need for an improved quality of life, rather than just longevity, as a therapeutic goal, has made the application of the human-animal bond in healthcare delivery a very desirable adjunctive therapy resource.

The proportion of elderly in this nation's population has increased faster than that of any other age group. The challenge of meeting the long-term healthcare needs of the elderly with cost-effective measures is enormous. Quality care is no longer equated to quantity care. The medical industry has started to embrace minimal or adequate care standards for economic and technological reasons. Animal facilitated therapy is perceived both as quality care and as beneficial to the entire patient-family-provider group (the holistic approach).

Stress Therapy

Animals have been utilized at multiple levels of the stress/grief process, often without the premeditation or even the realization needed to effectively facilitate the needed professional therapy. The potential roles of animals in the resolution of stress/grief include safety, companionship, nonjudgmental love, security, neutral communication topic, stress reduction, third-party triangulation, mood distraction, stabilization of the environment, physical detractors, reality anchors, or simply an alternative demand on the mental direction. The veterinary staff can benefit from any human-animal bond program, especially if trained as pet-by-prescription agents. Staff members used in these programs can experience improved self-esteem and feelings of worth that are seldom matched in daily activities. The placing of new pets in homes does bring in new clients, and the goodwill involvement often causes increased client referrals, but the real benefit of becoming involved in any animal facilitated therapy program is the personal healthcare team changes. The caring and sensitivity that overflows into the daily client relations within any delivery program makes all the difference in client retention and harmony.

Summary

Animal facilitated therapy has been labeled many things during the eight years since it was formally introduced as a treatment modality in the United States. In truth, animal facilitated therapy was used by the Army in convalescent centers in the United States during World War II. Regardless of labels, animal facilitated therapy is based on providing a source of warmth, compassion, and dignity for the stressed patient. This is also the definition of the hospice program as an alternative to acute care. Palliative care is based on patient dignity, and the interdisciplinary healthcare team that utilizes the human-animal bond as an adjunctive therapy quickly realizes its great benefits.

Any human–animal bond program is really people: the patient, the family, and the healthcare/support team. It is also the community it serves. Every program has realized the need for the support of the community and the support of volunteers. It also needs the skills of healthcare professionals who desire quality of life over quantity of care. The positive effects of the human-animal bond are substantial, but they are still only adjunctive to the efforts of the healthcare team, family, and patient. The "caring heart" pet therapist must be utilized by "caring heart" healthcare professionals if the new horizons in therapy are to be conquered.

References

CENSHARE. 1984. *Pet Connection.* Minneapolis: CENSHARE, University of Minnesota.

Delta Society, 289 Perimeter Road East, Renton, WA 98055-1329.

Fogle, B.M. 1981. *Interrelationships Between People and Pets.* Springfield, IL: Charles C. Thomas.

Honori, A., and A.M. Beck. (eds.) 1983. *New Perspectives on Our Lives with Companion Animals.* Philadelphia: University of Pennsylvania Press.

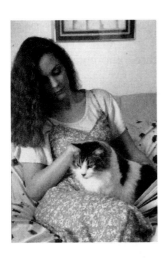

Appendix Q

Quality Care Promotions

PROMOTING HUMAN–ANIMAL bond programs means being a patient advocate, and being a patient advocate means speaking for the pet which cannot speak for itself. When speaking for another living entity, we cannot compromise on quality of veterinary healthcare delivery: that is a client's choice, not the choice of the veterinary practice. This appendix sample shows a few internal programs and potential promotions for the companion animal practice that wants to educate clients and improve the quality of life of its patients.

Specific Target Marketing

- Jan-Feb   Dental season (teeth graded 1+, 2+, 3+, 4+ for target marketing).
- Mar-Apr   Heartworm screening clinics.
                     Parasite and zoonotic prevention and control.
                     Cat concerns.
- May-Jun   National pet week theme expansion.
                     Puppy and kitten programs.
                     Traveling with your pet protection programs.
- Jul-Aug   Multi-pet "2-fur-1" care promotion.
                     Six-month, mid-year dental screening.
                     Breeder promotion.

- Sep-Oct   Over-40 programs for mature pets (anthropomorphic title, good in USA).
              Winterize your horse.
              Fall bathing promotional.
- Nov-Dec   Arthritis program.
              Lead II ECG cardiac screening program.

Internal Marketing Promotions

Below are several medical record documentation and internal promotion suggestions/options:

- Preferred client = fully vaccinated plus HW or FeLV plus annual fecal.
- Preanesthetic laboratory screening (PCV, TP, and BUN minimum).
- Sequential weight w/body score and other athletic programs.
- Postanesthetic acute pain killer injection.
- Full laboratory testing (FeLV, FIP, FIV, Lyme, etc.).
- Sequential laboratory testing to ensure wellness is restored.
- Eyes, ears, teeth, skin screening, and diagrams in records.
- Waivers, deferrals, and actions recorded in medical records.
- Three Rs (recall, recheck, remind) on *every* client before departure.
- "Other pets" screened with each visit.
- Proactive "refer a friend" effort by each staff member with each client.
- Technician nutrition/dental/parasite case follow-up.
- High communication desires:
  - Client handouts. These must be kept current, but also look at streamlining them at end of this year.
  - Pre-inpatient technician telephone call (24 hours ahead) to discuss fast/water intake needs.
  - Client calls by technician after anesthesia recovery; coordinate discharge time (with discharge instructions following phone call).
  - Client "thank you" for referral by reception staff (with new client newsletter).
  - Outpatient nurse does new client "thank you for picking us and are there any questions" 72 hours after visit.
  - Telephone receptionist does missed vaccination recall within 72 hours of expiration date, with "doctor and I" call (*"Doctor and I missed you and Fluffy this week, is everything okay at your house?"*).
- The New *Quality Care* Expectations
  - It is the growth of the practice, not the habits of the past.
  - It is the client coming through the door, not the hospital policies.
  - It is two "yes" alternatives, not a "no."
  - It is the patient advocacy, not the wallet size.
  - *Preferred clients* set the tone for levels of care, not the bottom 25 percent.

Preferred Clients

Preferred clients are ones who care as much as the practice staff does about the wellness of the animals. They show their concern by participating in the following practice programs:

• Annual doctor's consultation for total wellness care.
• Current on full vaccination program for each pet.
• Annual internal parasite exam (semi-annual in SE).
• Heartworm negative or FeLV negative.
• On year-round preventative (heartworm medicine or FeLV vaccination).
• Annual external parasite prevention program

Sample "Preferred Client" Pricing Schedule

Table Q.1. Sample vaccination program (one community example)

New Client**	Expired Protection Pet	Preferred Client*
$13.00	Rabies	$ 8.50
$22.50	K-9 Distemper Complex	$12.50
$16.50	Cat Distemper Complex	$11.50
$19.00	FeLV	$12.50

*Preferred client rates are set based on "media sensitivity" awareness levels in the community and on published VPI wellness reimbursement rates, not the closest veterinarian.
  • The doctor's consultation ($27.25) may be added to the above "preferred client participation programs" upon the preferred client's request.
  • *Phone narrative to make it happen:* Quality Care Animal Hospital, this is Gloria. How may we help you today?
    . . . **listen** . . . Vaccinations? I am glad you asked! Is your pet an established patient of ours?
    . . . **listen** . . . The doctor has looked at our good clients and noticed that we see them every three to four months. It seemed silly to us to do another "annual doctor's consultation" that close together, so we have changed our program for our *preferred clients.* We now offer our *preferred patients* a fast-in, fast-out, vaccination appointment with one of our nurses, Kathy or Karyn, for prices that are competitive even with the humane society! . . . On the other hand, if you have not seen doc in the past few months, or if you have concerns you want to discuss with a doctor, *then we need to schedule you for a full consultation,* . . . but we no longer make that decision for you about your pet care. . . . Which would you like to schedule today?
    . . . **listen** . . . Price for a full consultation? . . . It is over twice the length, with

the doctor and the nursing staff instead of the nursing staff only, so it is just over twice the price, about $60 instead of just over $20. . . . Which would you like to schedule today?

. . . listen . . .

**The new client fee schedule shown in Table Q.1 is based on the economic levels of the practices in the community and must be within 10 percent of the top of the market survey.

- Once a new client gets all services, a "big deal" is made of their automatically qualifying for the Preferred Client Program.
- If a client accesses a limited access "vaccination clinic," please ensure the staff lets the client know that "only a parasite exam and heartwrom (or FeLv) test and preventive" will qualify them for the "preferred client" rates.

Above all else, remember, at a quality care veterinary hospital, the staff sells only peace of mind; the client is allowed to buy all else, usually from two "yes" options.

DOOR HANGER VIA SCOUTS/CHURCH YOUTH/4-H/ETC.

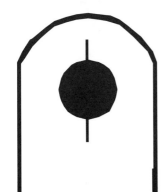

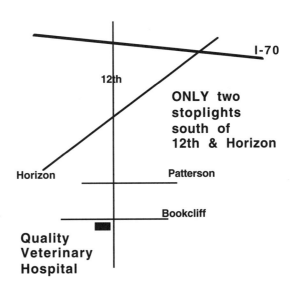

I-70

12th

**ONLY two
stoplights
south of
12th & Horizon**

Horizon

Patterson

Bookcliff

**Quality
Veterinary
Hospital**

HOSPITAL BENEFITS:

- Full-service Pet
  Healthcare

- Preferred Client
  Fast Access

- Seniors' Programs

- Major Credit Cards
  Accepted
- Walk-ins Welcomed

- Emergencies
  Anytime

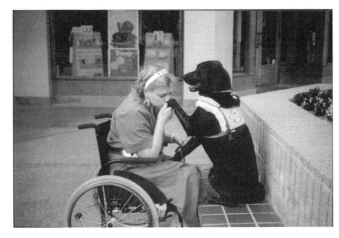

Appendix R

"Resale" Profit Center Museum: Potentials by Sharing Knowledge

Never miss an opportunity to raise the client's level of awareness.
—Dr. T.E. Catanzaro

IF WE are to believe recent merchandising seminars, the current trend toward a total merchandising approach has waned. There is some retail potential in a full-service veterinary hospital for companion animals, including exotics, but there is a greater potential within client education. There can be "special in-house services" for avian and exotic patients, including boarding and dietary management, and a retail display can call attention to this practice philosophy. Many facilities will have separate business endeavors for grooming and bathing, although they are usually accessed from the main healthcare facility. The boarding operations can be marketed as a "pet hotel," a "pet resort," a "critter camp", a "pet bed and breakfast", or even a "pet vacationland," depending upon the decor and marketing philosophy. Some will be either co-located or in close proximity to the groomer, who therefore acts as the boarding manager. The professional staff of current practices should have provisions for both behavior training and bereavement counseling for clients. A pet boutique can be established instead of the standard "retail area." It could sell quality antiques and collectibles pertaining to animal and pet related supplies. The "customer service" area of the practice could include multiple lines of nutritional products, pet toys, cages, training halters and collars, gifts, treats, leashes, and even "how to" books. Real entrepreneurs have built pet complexes around a central parking area and sublet the separate entities to others, collecting rent while capitalizing on the one-stop shopping desires of the current generation. But these "new trends" are now old and have been diluted by the pet super stores, so these traditional ideas are not for all of us.

An Alternative

The veterinarian who graduated in the days of practitioner shortages, if you can remember that long ago, has a different problem. In those "good old days" it was unethical to board, groom, have displays, or even have bulletin boards for client information exchanges. It must have been something like Prohibition, but for veterinarians only. The goal today is to meet the clients' needs while being a patient advocate. This "charter" is often evaluated by the ability to sleep at night or look in the mirror, which is not always easy for those colleagues who merchandise as if they were discount stores.

The concept of a museum showcase has been around for quite awhile, yet most of those display jars have been put on some back shelf. Consider presenting the following type of museum in your reception area. Display a flea under a lens, with a label indicating the average reproductive potential if gone untreated. Behind the flea place a line of your flea products, labeled as to their efficacy in stopping the flea life cycle, with a note to ask anyone on the staff for details. Or display that jar of roundworms, with a label indicating the possibility for environmental contamination (larval migrans); place a Fecalizer/Ovassy next to it, with a note stating, "Our veterinarian recommends stool samples be submitted twice a year to prevent these from occurring in your pet's intestinal track or in your family." Can you think of which Iams/Hill's Diets you would display behind the kidney stones and what the card would say? I shouldn't need to discuss the potential of the Merial rubber heartworm model (with the new medications which treat these zoonotic threats to the family) or the model of a teeth arcade, or what to put behind those models.

Other items also can be interspersed in the museum; these might include a bottle of Mycodex with Carbaryl, with a simple note saying, "A good flea shampoo and great for white coat dogs"; a bottle of Nutriderm that has a note saying, "Needed for glossy coats if you pet is fed exclusively dry food"; or even a bottle of Pet Tabs with a note that says, "Good for pregnant or lactating dogs." This subtle merchandising in the museum should be in the reception room if your clients usually have to wait. It will usually create examination room discussions, and that is where the client is "allowed to buy" what they noticed and discussed with the doctor. A museum display is designed not to "sell," but to educate. The only thing we should "sell" in veterinary healthcare delivery is "peace of mind" for the client. All else, clients are "allowed to buy," preferably from two "yes" options advocated by a caring veterinary professional.

Some management "experts" advocate a "point of purchase display" near the discharge area. This sounds nice, but watch your clients. When they leave the examination room, they want to leave. Impulse buys are not on their minds or in their traffic patterns; impulse buying is not a healthcare user characteristic. Clients seldom wait and browse, even if the reception area is inefficient and they are made to wait to "settle the bill." As a point of interest, never put a price on the actual product itself (á la the grocery store). Instead, put the price on the card that accompanies the product or on the shelf front under the product. Not only is this easier for your staff when prices change, but when clients go to replace products, there are no old prices on the containers to remind them of the previous price, or the current inflationary mark-ups.

Do It in a Unique Way

Dr. Eppinger, in the mountain town of Nederland, Colorado, developed her museum around some antiques from the local community. Clients are drawn to her shadow box. What if the display had folklore and explanations (e.g., "When fleas leave your body, you are about to die.")? Got your interest about fleas? Fleas are very sensitive to body temperature changes and will leave a body with a high fever. It's a very simple explanation, but it gets the client to stop and look at the display. There are many folklore stories, and most are founded in fact. Most clients like to know more about the folklore, and it helps to keep them interested when times are busy.

While the museum concept often defeats the merchandising strategy of letting the client touch the product, it does do what the traditional discount-store stacks do not. It informs and educates the client. That makes it a client service. Our clients are not customers; they are guests, and they deserve the quality hospitality expected in a caring and concerned healthcare facility. American consumers are trained to the mantra "buyer beware," but our clients trust our professional charge to care for the creatures of the earth, and they should not be abused by a quantity-sale work ethic. Innovative merchandising can be fun and tailored to our respective practice styles. Just remember our professional and ethical charge to provide a client service first.

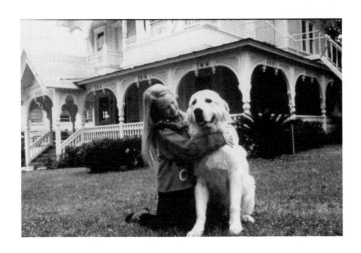

Appendix S

Pain Scoring

CLIENTS DO not want their pets to be in pain, and staff hates to see an animal in pain. How do you get awareness in your practice about pain management so the human-animal bond does not get stressed? Establish a pain scoring system where everyone participates every day! No patient goes unscored during any trauma presentation, and inpatients are minimally tracked for changes on a t.i.d. basis.

We endorse the pain scoring system that was described in the *Compendium on Continuing Education for the Practicing Veterinarian* (February 1998, 140–153); the eight factors with 0–3 scoring for each factor constitute the most thorough assessment tool available. However, some practices like a simpler system, so here is a "10 count and you are out" system. All pain scored 2 or higher should have intervention, and the practice protocol *cannot* override a pain score by a staff member!

Of course, the clinician must make a medical determination on the exact pain medication used, but here are some guidelines that are widely accepted:

- *Lower scores:* torbutrol +/- Acepromazine, rimadyl, Ascriptin, Fledene, Phenylbutazone.
- *Moderate scores:* Codeine, Ketoprofin.
- *Higher scores:* Fentanyl patch, Oxymorphone, Morphine, spinal injection.

Table S.1. Simple pain scoring system

Pain Score	Description
P-0	No pain
P-1	Maybe there was pain
P-2	There should be pain (minor wounds, pro-op dental, abrasions, etc.)
P-3	Post-op soft tissue surgery or more extensive wounds
P-4	Extractions or more extensive dental procedures
P-5	Multiple extractions, carnasal extractions
P-6	Declaw, post-op cruciate, fracture, blunt abdominal trauma
P-7	Head pressing attitude
P-8	Major soft-tissue wound, severe fracture, pancreatitis
P-9	Extensive burns, multiple fractures, spinal trauma, septic gut, eye injury
P-10	Patient SCREAMING!

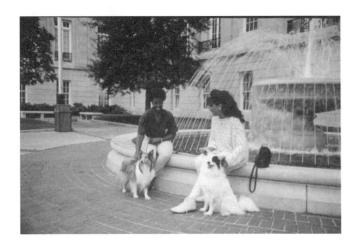

Appendix T

Traveling Pets

OVER HALF of Americans took their dogs with them on vacation in 1999. Most veterinarians appear *not* to care. They do not ask about pet travel, either with new clients or with existing clients. This is called, *not bonding* with your clients. Ask yourself these questions:

- Did I ask the new client where the pet geographically came from?
- Did I ask about current vacation plans and the pet's destiny?
- What do I know about valley fever (important for "snow bird" clients)?
- What do I know about Lyme disease incidence in other areas?
- What do I know about asymptomatic giardiasis (beaver fever)?
- What do I know about salmon disease, if the client travels to the Northwest?
- What should I do for Bordetella with traveling pets?
- What are the tularemia (rabbit fever) dangers for hunting dogs?
- Did I tell my clients about the parasite prevention portion of the new heartworm preventatives?
- Have I discussed the strategic deworming protocols of the CDC web site with my clients?
- What are the current medication protocols for motion sickness?
- What are the preferred tranquilization methods for traveling cats or dogs?

We have always recommended that a veterinary practice create a flyer about local precautions against the threats and dangers of parasites and diseases of the community and provide it to their new clients. Now we recommend that the caring veterinary practice create a flyer that covers "traveling with your pet" precautions, addressing the national threats and dangers of parasites and diseases common in other areas of this country. Brochure-building information can be found in *Building the Successful Veterinary Practice* (Volume 3); send your staff into the fray to build a client-friendly information booklet/flyer.

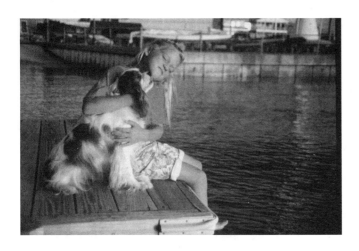

Appendix U

Dental Scoring and Contesting

Dental grades only are required for patients with teeth.
—Dr. T.E. Cantanzaro

Scoring

THE HUMAN–ANIMAL bond is stressed when "puppy kisses" get to the point where the smell will gag the owner. Brown teeth mean bad breath, and red gums mean pain; to not do anything means *you don't care!* Wanting to "restore puppy kisses" is a nice phrase to use when opening the discussion about dental care.

We know that very few pet owners like the toothpaste route (look at the toothpaste refill rate). We must add excitement to the process, so we often ask our client's staff to participate in a "puppy kiss" contest. To start a contest, everyone must know the rules, and they are not difficult, but it requires a total commitment by everyone to "make it happen," here are the basics:

• *Brown Teeth = Bad Breath* and *Red Gums = Pain.* The client needs to hear this loud and clear; if the client's mouth looked like his/her pet's mouth, he/she would have *no friends.*
• The CET brochure and the new Upjohn flyer have four sequential pictures, from

red gums (grade 1, +, or 1+), to brown teeth without much plaque (grade 2, ++, or 2+), to heavy plaque (grade 3, +++, or 3+), to bone destruction (grade 4, ++++, or 4+).

- The dental grade will be recorded during each visit, but only *after* looking at the previous grading level.
- In progressive practices, the dental grade will be followed by a box "❏". A box ❏ denotes a "need" stated to the client.
- In a high communication practice, the entry in the box (need = ❏) is the client's response to the stated need: W = waiver (get out of my face), D = defer (maybe next time), A = appointment (after payday), or X = do it now!
- Every time a "need box" ❏ has something besides an "X" in it, it will be followed by the provider's response: 3w = three weeks, 4m = four months, etc.
- Each encounter with a client/patient requires the next contact (the three Rs) be established before the client departs the practice, done *today*, without exception: recall (phone), remind (mail), or recheck (come back in).
- The dental grade and three R expectations are entered into the computer service code (recall) system during the invoicing process.

This sets the system for the next phase, which is internal marketing. The AAHA dental tapes and Upjohn dental booklets are good training aids if used by the entire healthcare delivery team, including, but not limited to, doctors, nurses, dental hygiene technicians, receptionists, etc. Please remember two things: (1) effective internal marketing *starts* with training, and (2) your first and most important client is the staff member.

As an example, with effective training, for the *recall* or *recheck,* either a "❏ 3w" or "❏ 3w" causes the same team and computer expectation: a first week, nightly garlic water (tuna water for cats) tooth rub for the dog (they like the flavor); a second week using "baking soda in the garlic water" for the nightly tooth rub, to introduce the abrasion feeling; a third week using "a cloth with the baking soda garlic water" for the nightly tooth rub, so the pets get used to a foreign body in their mouths. After the clients do this "no cost" test, they are told to return in three weeks for a courtesy dental hygiene consult with the dental hygiene technician. The result is generally impressive; the request rate for the hospital to clean the pet's teeth is over a 50 percent (most practices are closer to 75 percent). Clients are tired of playing with the mouth.

For the *remind,* we must use the dental grade to establish the postcard narrative to remind the client where the discussions were during the last veterinary encounter, for example:

- 1+ = "The last time you and White Fang were in, we talked about (his/her) red gums and pain. Please check and see if this is resolved. If not, please schedule a consult with our dental hygiene technician; it is a courtesy visit this time because we are concerned about the potential pain as well as the bad breath."
- 2+ = "The last time you and White Fang were in, we talked about (his/her) brown teeth and bad breath. Please check and see if this is improving. If not,

please schedule a consult with our dental hygiene technician; it is a courtesy visit this time because we are concerned about the bad breath as well as potential infections."

- 3+ = "The last time you and White Fang were in, we talked about (his/her) bad plaque, infection, and the terrible breath. Please check and see if this has gotten worse. If you can, please schedule a consult with our dental hygiene technician; it is a courtesy visit this time because, in addition to the bad breath, we are concerned about your pets shortened life span when teeth get this bad."
- 4+ = "The last time you and White Fang were in, we talked about the generalized infection and major health hazard caused by teeth. Please schedule a consult with our dental hygiene technician; it is a courtesy visit this time because we are concerned about the shortened life span, complicating problems, and terrible breath caused by this bad a mouth."

The narratives need to be tailored to the providers in *your* practice, because they need to match the discussion phrases of the examination room as well as those of the dental hygiene technicians and receptionists. They are specific to *your* practice philosophy. We considered both Grade 3+ and Grade 4+ to be "oral surgery," and they are listed as such on the invoices.

So "On with the Contest"

The key to making a new project fun is to be innovative. Many practices use "contesting" as a way to make "practice emphasis" a fun time for all. As reported in *AAHA Trends* "Featured Practice," this "contesting" concept has been used very effectively by Dr. Connie Moll at Midland Animal Clinic, Midland, Michigan.

The concept is simply to bring the staff's attention to bear on a program of interest and share the reward of the effort. This has been called the GMP (greatest management principle) by Michael LeBoeuf (1989) a wonderful and easy reading paperback text); *behavior rewarded is behavior that will be repeated.* In the greater scheme of things, contesting costs money, and the contest "prizes" require taxes to be paid on the awards. The flip side of this "expense" is the value-added benefit derived when the staff "buy" the program and become promoters rather than observers.

Not all practices can use contesting effectively; it is participant dependent. When a bonus or productivity pay is awarded with an employer's comment, "this is costing me money," its positive effects are erased immediately. Contesting and productivity pay systems are based on exceeding realistic expectations. I say realistic expectations because to be effective, at least 60 percent of the staff needs to "win." This means the "program" stretch must be incremental: small steps are required to allow repetitive successes.

If contesting seems an interesting concept for your practice, the attached chart is offered as a diagrammatic representation of a contesting effort. The program of interest does not have to be dentals nor does the owner have to take a vacation, but these are the things that excited the practice that requested we develop the picture for them to follow. The choice is yours, share success or share mediocrity; the world will keep turning regardless.

References

LeBoeuf, M. 1989. *The Greatest Management Principle in the World.* Berkeley Publishing Group.

DENTAL CONTEST PLAN

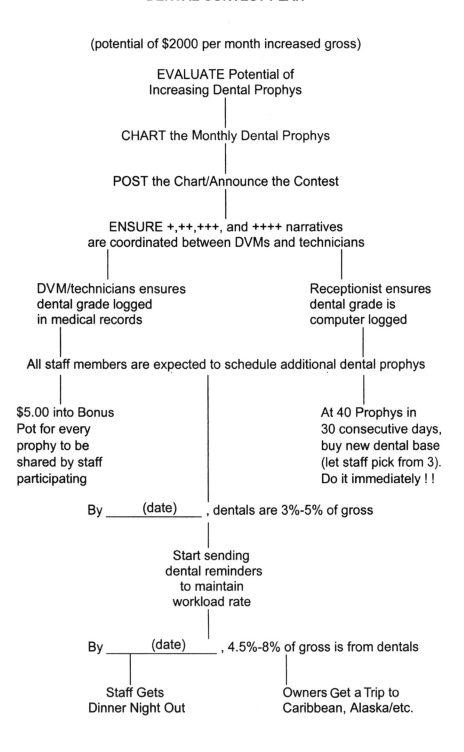

(potential of $2000 per month increased gross)

EVALUATE Potential of
Increasing Dental Prophys

CHART the Monthly Dental Prophys

POST the Chart/Announce the Contest

ENSURE +,++,+++, and ++++ narratives
are coordinated between DVMs and technicians

DVM/technicians ensures
dental grade logged
in medical records

Receptionist ensures
dental grade is
computer logged

All staff members are expected to schedule additional dental prophys

$5.00 into Bonus
Pot for every
prophy to be
shared by staff
participating

At 40 Prophys in
30 consecutive days,
buy new dental base
(let staff pick from 3).
Do it immediately ! !

By _____(date)_____ , dentals are 3%-5% of gross

Start sending
dental reminders
to maintain
workload rate

By _____(date)_____ , 4.5%-8% of gross is from dentals

Staff Gets
Dinner Night Out

Owners Get a Trip to
Caribbean, Alaska/etc.

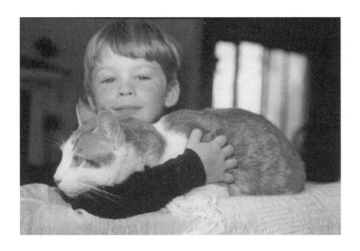

Appendix V

Body Scoring and Nutritional Scoring

Body Scoring

FOR YEARS, the veterinary profession has been selling pet food, but only recently have we actually begun the active role of wellness counselors. Most practices try to take sequential weights, but have not developed an easy system to record the assessment of that weight; we call this documentation *body scoring*. Hill's and Pfizer have offered five-point systems, and Purina has provided a nine-point system; use the one that excites your doctors and staff. In the act of body scoring, the veterinary staff member assumes an active role in evaluating the overall condition of the pet, since there are a significant number of obese and malnourished pets in the general population. As a general rule, every pet's body score should be recorded at each visit following the weight (e.g., 35/5).

Just as with the pain scoring model, the staff member must be trained to make a judgment about the course of action necessary to address the nutritional condition; vendors have more than ample systems, just ensure there is a single standard in your practice so clients do not get confused. According to clinical experts, any patient with a score of 3 or below is probably in need of immediate intervention to prevent death. Likewise, animals with a score of 7 or higher need an immediate response to their condition to prevent life-altering disease or conditions.

Table V.1. Nine-point body scoring system

Score	Description
x1	Animal abuse/neglect—Violation of Title 9, CFR
W-2	Moderate malnourishment—Ribs and bones visibly pronounced, marked muscle loss throughout the body.
W-3	Early malnourishment—Ribs pronounced and visible, slight degree of muscle loss in parts of the body.
W-4	Slightly thin—Ribs visible through skin, but does not exhibit gross muscle loss in the rest of the body.
W-5	Ideal Condition—Good muscle tone, ribs not visible through skin, but able to palpate individual ribs without effort.
W-6	Slightly obese—Ribs not visible, but still palpable with less definition.
W-7	Moderately obese—Cannot feel individual ribs upon palpation, animal will probably fatigue quickly with exercise.
W-8	Severely obese—Cannot feel individual ribs upon palpation, animal has difficulty with exercise.
W-9	Morbidly obese—Animal has difficulty walking, moving or breathing.
N-3	Anorexia for one (1) day

Hill's and Pfizer provide aids which recommend a five-point system that can be used for dogs and cats (if the doctors or staff start using decimals, e.g. 4.5, shift to the nine-point system and do not allow decimals).

- Body condition score of 1 = Very thin
- Body condition score of 2 = Underweight
- Body condition score of 3 = Ideal
- Body condition score of 4 = Overweight
- Body condition score of 5 = Obese

Nutritional Scoring

Body scoring of the well pet often leads into nutritional scoring of the inpatient animal. There has been some excellent literature from the Veterinary Emergency and Critical Care Society on the importance of nutritional supplementation for ill pets, and like pain scoring, it should be an "all staff" patient advocacy program within the practice. It is critical that every member of the team be accountable for monitoring every inpatient with each feeding; some hospital directors have set the standard that nutritional scoring is performed on each patient at least twice a day while they are in the hospital since recovery is so dependent on the metabolic process.

Just as with the pain scoring model, the clinician must make a professional judgment about the course of action necessary to address the nutritional deficiency. According to clinical experts, any patient with a score of 4 or higher needs

Table V.2. Inpatient nutritional scoring

Score	Description
N-0	History of eating well
N-1	Off feed, eating, history of slow eating in cage
N-2	Purposeful NPO
N-3	Anorexia for one (1) day
N-4	Anorexia for two (2) days
N-5	Anorexia for three (3) days
N-6	Anorexia for four (4) days
N-7	Anorexia for five (5) days

These scores should be modified in the event of disease, injury, or other stresses:

Add 1	In cases of mild disease, injury, or surgery
Add 2	In cases of moderate/febrile disease, injury, or surgery
Add 3	In cases of severe disease, injury, or surgery

an immediate response to the nutritional deficiency. This response may be as simple as hand feeding or low-dose oral glucose for enterokinetic maintenance. In cases where the patient's response is mediated, the placement of a nasogastric tube may be required for administration of glucose, Clinicare or a/d gruel. If the duration of the treatment is anticipated to be prolonged, the placement of a pharyngostomy or PEG tube may be indicated.

Body scoring and nutritional scoring, like pain scoring, are methods for *internal* healthcare communications, not numbers for clients. Clients must hear the words and the explanations. Clients must be able to picture the outcome of neglect, and the rewards of appropriate care, for the animals for which they have assumed accountability. Remember the three basic rules of ensuring the client perceives quality veterinary healthcare delivery:

- **Never allow pain.**
- **Never allow puking.**
- **Help the client find ways to feed his/her animal.**

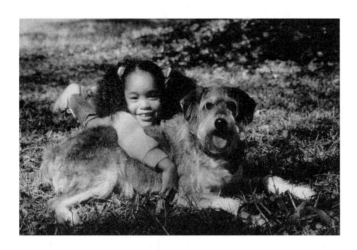

Appendix W

Marketing Nutritional Wellness

There is no overhead involved in something which replaces "coffee time."
—Dr. T.E. Catanzaro

FOR YEARS, we have thought things like grooming have no net, nutritional sales have minimal net, and we are professionals and do not "sell." These types of functions were even "unethical" a decade ago. The times have changed, and the companion animal veterinary profession has polarized into two camps: (1) change and capitalize upon the new opportunities and (2) maintain what we have always done, and "this, too, shall pass." The latter thought has caused practices to decrease their liquidity.

Before we start, let me state that I am *not* a believer in sales! I believe in letting clients buy and in providing them with options. Marketing is a three-step alignment process: (1) alerting a client to a preexisting need of the pet and elevating that to a want, (2) making the client aware that our profession now has some alternatives to meet the need and assuring the client that our own scope of services can meet it, and (3) taking a few moments to validate the client's decision, regardless of the choice made, and setting a time to "make it happen." In today's environment, marketing is the ability to believe in what you do and let others know that it is worthwhile. See *Veterinary Healthcare Services: Options in Delivery* (2000) for a more detailed explanation of the entire alignment process.

Nutrition as a Profit Center

Nutritional wellness is a contemporary healthcare concern (see Catanzaro 1989). *Wellness* is a popular term for our clients in their own healthcare and nutritional counseling and is well accepted for people. In addition, nutritional wellness is a media industry in itself. The phrase *nutritional wellness* brings mental images into our clients' minds that makes our marketing efforts easier. The sad thing to note is that Hill's research shows that while most practices have started 30 percent or more of their patients on some form of quality diet, less than 7 percent of the patients stay on for an entire year; we are not doing our job as patient advocates when this many animals are allowed to "fall off" a quality nutritional program.

There are those who have started to sell nutritional products, and there are those who have recently stopped selling maintenance diets because of the "pet food warehouse" competition in their catchment area(s). Regardless of the decision, there is one important "profit center" concept to understand: *your practice overhead is a fixed cost whenever you consider adding any new line item.*

For years, we considered square footage and other apportionment methods to determine profitability of a service or product, but in this decade that thought pattern is outmoded. In the cost-benefit analysis, if the service or product replaces something else, the value of each must be assessed and compared. If the new line item or service only replaces idle time ("coffee time"), there is no overhead expense. You would pay the overhead expenses with or without the new product line or service. This is the category in which I usually find pet food and nutritional counseling. It is a spare time activity within a practice, not displacing anything else.

Rules of Thumb

Rule 1. In this day of veterinary diversification, marketing of nutritional products has become a concern in many practices. The current rule of thumb is that when the income from pet food exceeds 3 percent of gross, it should become a separate expense element and be managed as its own profit center. The standard markup on pet food makes volume a tracking concern if the lower net is combined into the drug and medical supply account. To see pet food as a profit center, rather than just a client service, it needs to be tracked separately.

Rule 2. The rule of thumb that prices are often set by our competitors has waned. The new rule of thumb is, "Prices are controlled by the most efficient agency known; the consumer" (*Fortune Magazine,* April 5, 1993). This is especially true when competing in this market, since the pet or feed stores carry similar products and the manufacturers' marketing efforts are aimed at the product and not the outlet. The emerging pet food warehouses have a volume discount capability seldom matched by a veterinary practice complex. This is a fact and should not be confused with something a practice can change.

Rule 3. The rule of thumb that a veterinarian is worth in excess of $220 per hour in the examination room or surgical suite makes nutritional counseling by the veterinarian a low-payoff activity, if nutritional counseling replaces professional healthcare. If it replaces coffee time, it is not a comparison issue. The wages a practice usually pays the paraprofessional staff make their nutritional counseling efforts a higher payoff practice activity.

Rule 4. The last rule of thumb is the medical basis of this discussion. Is nutrition important to health? Does every animal deserve to be on a nutritionally complete and balanced diet? Is digestibility also a concern? How would you prefer a pet owner to receive information concerning nutrition when it must fit into the veterinary healthcare delivery plan? Do you want your practice to control the veterinary healthcare delivery plan? If most of the answers are yes, the rule of thumb is, "Provide it or lose it."

Managing Public Perception

Clients must believe in what we tell them. To be professional and believable, we must sincerely and medically endorse whatever we are saying. Marketing pet food without believing in the product usually results in the practice effort becoming a cost center rather than a profit center. The professional training of our staff, and ourselves, includes the mental attitude adjustments required to develop nutritional counseling as a needed service as well as a profit center. In one Illinois practice, when the doctors were asked what they fed to their own animals, only two of the six were feeding premium diets. We made a pact; everyone would feed only "practice available" diets for 90 days (even if they had to be sold at cost to the staff). At the end of the 90 days, retail nutritional product sales had increased by 19 percent. The team saw the difference, believed in the products, and naturally started to share their belief in their nutritional quality with the clients.

Discuss with your staff why certain diets are indicated, why Iams or Hill's or ProPlan or Waltham, or whatever you stock, is available in your practice, and why you professionally feel certain animals need specific dietary management. Get the staff to believe in what you believe. More important, at the end of each month, ask each paraprofessional the following three questions:

1. How many clients were referred to you (the veterinary nutritional advisor) this month (by veterinarian, if applicable)?

2. What is the number of active nutritional patients (contacted within the past 30 days) being tracked by each veterinary nutritional advisor as of the end of each month?

3. How many nutritional patients did you bring in for "return weigh-ins" during the past month (by veterinary nutritional advisor, if applicable)?

4. How many patients were provided sequential laboratory screens of body chemistry levels to ensure the feeding trial is/was effective?

These questions are designed to *empower* the veterinary nutritional advisor, based on training completed outside or inside the practice. They are designed to show the practice's confidence in the capability of the staff member to follow his/her "own clients" and delegate the client counseling to a cost effective level within the practice. The questions utilized are in concert with the values of most paraprofessionals: client service and a caring approach to wellness. They center on factors for which the staff member has *complete accountability.* If revenue dollars are brought into the equation, excuses are possible (over the counter sales, size of purchases, cross sales, etc.). This would be detrimental to measuring personal success.

In cases of tracking client access, the paraprofessional can be *proud* of the service provided. In healthcare delivery, it has been shown that *staff pride* is perceived by the client as *quality.* Caring and belief in the value-based quality received promote client bonding. And bonding is what causes return trade (and increased liquidity).

Each client has specific "hot buttons," those things that really spark an interest or keep the client's attention. The receptionist, the technician, and the veterinarian need to become a team in writing those key personal elements in some specific area of the medical record. This allows more effective communication with the client since analogies can be drawn. The marathon runner will usually understand the need for stamina; the nurse will understand the need for a balanced nutritional program; or a parent will generally understand the need for an owner to provide a nutritionally complete diet for animals under their care. Inversely, the overweight client will generally not respond favorably to statements about a *fat pet,* but may respond to a comment about the need for higher fiber and extended life span, while the client who likes to feed table scraps and rebels when we recommend stopping will often respond to the wellness need when we point out that a nutritional consultation can balance the diet to a point where a few specific table scraps are okay during the transition to a better lifestyle and fitness state for the pet.

The public perception of nutritional wellness is formed by many factors, most of which are out of the veterinarian's control. The local media intensity of human nutritional center advertising programs will pre-sensitize the client. The family standards for balanced or complete diets will affect the perception of importance of diet for the pet. The amount of junk food consumed in the client's daily lifestyle will affect the importance of a controlled diet in his/her pet's life. The veterinary practice staff cannot affect these environmental factors to any significant degree.

Making It Happen in Your Practice

The total patient advocacy program of your practice style will allow nutritional counseling to be seen as a farce or as a sincere concern. How you approach the healthcare needs of the pet from the first visit will often set the stage for nutritional counseling. Client education in the areas of vaccinations, internal and external parasite screens, preanesthesia laboratory testing, documented physical examinations, dental hygiene exams, and similar routine healthcare concerns make the use of nutritional counseling seem normal.

The veterinarian must set the stage for the need, but does not have to conduct the nutritional counseling. A well-trained technician or receptionist can act as the nutritional advisor. In this role, the technician or receptionist acts as an extender for the veterinarians within the practice. Veterinary extenders (both people and things) are needed in every practice: they allow the veterinarians to stay in the examination room or surgical suite and earn the high income that they were trained to earn.

The statement, "Fluffy seems a little heavy. Let's get you with our nutritional counselor and see if we can work out a system that will help with this challenge," conveys a depth of expertise within the practice. It also indicates that the veterinarian trusts the judgment of the staff member, which makes it necessary that standards be discussed and understood before the first internal referral to one of our veterinary extenders occurs. The referral also establishes that veterinary extender as a care provider and makes that person responsible for a portion of the healthcare follow-up, that portion which pertains to nutritional wellness.

One examination room can often be set up for routine use by the trained staff, with certificates of training and other credentials hanging on the walls for the clients to read. The display of these "glory walls" should not be restricted to the veterinarians on staff. These displays lend an important credibility and recognition to our support staff. To a veterinary extender who serves as a nutritional counselor, the scale is an important instrument and should reflect a professional approach to monitoring weight loss or gain. Holding animals while standing on a bathroom scale is not the image we want. An appropriate floor scale could be considered as a veterinary extender since it saves manpower time.

The routine follow-up weighing of animals on nutritional programs is expected and can easily be programmed for a veterinary extender to monitor, including recall reminders if the pet fails to appear for monitoring. The fact that the nutritional counselor monitors the weigh-ins does not require that the recall be done by that trained person. Any member of the staff can be trained to make "Doctor and I" recalls. For example, after the appropriate phone introduction is made, say, "The doctor and I have noted that we didn't get to weigh Fluffy this month. Is everything okay with you and Fluffy?". This form of client and patient advocacy by the veterinary extenders will be perceived by most clients as professional caring, making the next practice visit that much more pleasant.

To balance the marketing of nutritional products with the sincere caring that is expected in quality practices, some cases will not need pet food. There are certain breeds that can eat any commercial diet and maintain good health, while others gain weight or may become deficient in some portion of their nutritional requirements. A well-trained nutritional counselor will know when to supplement, when to change feeds, and when to use the "grain of common sense" and just try to delete a portion of the table scraps from the diet.

Service has been defined as adding people to the product. *Profit* is adding any net income to some action, void, or habit which had none. Marketing nutritional wellness fits these definitions exceptionally well, especially when we consider using the internally trained veterinary extender as the means to make it happen.

References

Catanzaro, T.E. 1989. How to Market Nutritional Wellness—Use Practice Extenders to Stretch Your Influence. *Veterinary Forum* (March).

Catanzaro, T.E., T. Haig, P. Weinstein, J. Leake, and H. Howell. 2000. *Veterinary Healthcare Services: Options in Delivery*. Ames: Iowa State University Press.

Huey, J. 1993. Managing in the Midst of Chaos. *Fortune Magazine* (April 5).

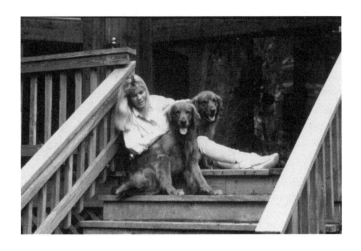

Appendix X

Radiology/Imaging Programs: Imaging Is a Bonding Activity

THE HUMAN–ANIMAL bond is based on the premise that stewards of other living things want to do what is best for their wards. For some reason, this premise is most violated in veterinary imaging: "tincture of time" does not do anyone any good, yet it is a common delaying tactic in many veterinary facilities! The following observations should be assessed in a team meeting:

- Limping animals deserve X rays *before* we determine that we can treat the ailment medically.
- Moist rales need radiographic assessment.
- Chronic gut syndrome deserves an imaging assessment.
- The early root defects that begin to appear in late Grade 2+ teeth can only be assessed by reviewing X rays of the roots.
- The "over 40" consultation should include a physical assessment that incorporates thoracic and abdominal screen radiographs.
- Ultrasound is not a gimmick; it is an imaging system that requires a highly skilled professional to interpret it.

- Endoscopy has its place: in the colon, in the joint, and in other locations other than the storage closet.
- Many hollow body organs need either contrast radiography or ultrasound for proper physiological assessment, and palpation is not that sensitive!
- Penn-Hip has it's place in the early diagnosis of orthopedic conditions, but is not a "cure all"; practices using the Penn-Hip have increased their imaging from knowledge, not from publicity.
- The automatic processor will usually cause a 30 percent income/utilization increase in imaging procedures over the hand tanks and also provides a dry film in a safer atmosphere.

One of the easiest techniques we have used for practices that want to change their imaging habits is to first have the entire veterinary practice team write a "job description" for the X-ray machine, then have them commit to use it for the appropriate tasks.

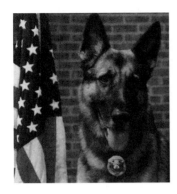

Appendix Y

Why Animal Welfare Is Important to Your Image

FOR THE record, I am not an extremist, I am not a bleeding heart, and I am not a passing consultant. As a veterinarian, I have been doing animal abuse and neglect interactions with law enforcement agencies around the world for over 25 years. I am a charter member of both the Delta Society and the American Association of Human-Animal Bond Veterinarians; I am also a current Board member of Vet One. I sincerely believe that the term "animal rights" is a forensic term, not nature's way. If it were nature's way, we could put a coyote and a rabbit in a 10 x 10 room for an hour, and half the time the rabbit would come out picking it's teeth; that is not the way of life.

The Rights of Animals

Animal rights are an essential element of civilized society, but they are the laws of a community, not nature. The original Animal Welfare Act was written to protect animals at draft, and it was soon applied to the sweat shops abusing children. The actual implementation provisions are updated annually in Chapter 1, Title 9, Code of Federal Regulations (CFR), and should be in every veterinary practice library as an operational resource. While these regulations are legally written for animals on display and animals during interstate movement, they provide minimum essential husbandry requirements for most common species.

Care of Animals

> *The animal should not show: trauma, stress, overheating, excessive cooling, behavioral stress, physical harm, or unnecessary discomfort.*
>
> *Deprivation of food or water shall not be used to train, work, or otherwise handle animals . . . animals will receive full dietary and nutritional requirements each day.*
>
> *An animal shall not be subjected to any combination of temperature, humidity, and time that is detrimental to the animal's health or well-being.*
>
> *—Title 9, CH 1, Sec 2.131*

As a veterinarian, we each know what is normal and what is abnormal. We usually know what is caused by disease and what is caused by husbandry. We have the ability to act as professionals in animal neglect because we know what is normal. An animal that is not normal has been neglected, sometimes covertly and other times overtly, but neglect is simply, "That animal is not being treated right." The proof of abuse requires an intent, which is the role of investigators, not the veterinarian. What is most important to remember is that there is a 95 percent correlation between animal abuse and child abuse (UK research, Delta Society proceedings), and to allow an animal abuse case to go unreported is to put some child in potential jeopardy!

Talking to the Client

The extracts from Title 9, Code of Federal Regulations, are just that. They provide veterinary healthcare professionals a baseline for using their professional opinion with confidence. Legally, Title 9, CFR, applies to animals on display, those undergoing interstate shipment, or critters used in research; they are extensive and have provisions for most species, although I have extracted only a few of the cat and dog provisions for illustration. When the Animal Welfare Act, a federal law, is annually translated into the CFR, many "common sense" elements are defined, which provides law enforcement officials, kennel staff, humane organizations, and animal owners a degree of confidence when listening to a veterinary healthcare professional's opinion on animal neglect or abuse.

Humane Handling, Care, Treatment of Dogs and Cats

> *Dogs and cats must be provided adequate shelter from the elements at all times to protect their health and well-being. Housing must be designed and constructed so they are structurally sound, kept in good repair, made of materials that are readily cleaned and sanitized, and protect the animal from injury, contain the animal(s) securely, and restrict other animals from entering.*
>
> *Cleaning—hard surfaces must be spot-cleaned daily and sanitized, and floors must be spot-cleaned with sufficient frequency to ensure all the freedom to avoid contact with excreta.*
>
> *Ambient temperatures in the facility, or traveling housing, must not drop below 50°F for dogs and cats not acclimated to lower temperatures, nor rise above 85°F, for more than 4 consecutive hours, except as approved by a veterinarian.*
>
> *Cats over 4.4 kg (8.8 lbs) must be provided with at least 4.0 ft² (exclusive of*

> *food or water pans), and be at least 24 inches high. No more than 12 cats are allowed in a single primary enclosure.*
>
> *Each dog must be provided with floor space calculated at least as: mathematical square of the sum of the length of the dog in inches (measured from base of tail to tip of nose) plus 6 inches, then divided by 144 to get square feet, with a height 6 inches higher than the head of the tallest dog in the facility, when in a standing position. No more than 12 dogs are allowed in a single primary enclosure.*
>
> *Dogs and cats must be fed at last once daily; food must be uncontaminated, wholesome, palatable, and of sufficient quantity and nutritive value to maintain the normal condition and weight of the animal. If potable water is not continually available, it must be offered not less than twice a day for at least one hour each time.*
>
> *An effective program for control of insects and external parasites must be established and maintained as to promote the health and well-being of the animals and reduce contamination by pests (includes other birds or mammals).*
>
> *—Title 9, CFR, CH 1, Part 3, Subpart A*
> *(extracted elements)*

It is important to understand that while over 75 percent of companion animals are considered family members, the law provides that animals are "owned property." The real challenge lies in the simple fact that people learn pet ownership from the same people who were their parents, and the famous quote is, "When I have kids, I am not raising them the way I was raised!" Most parents do not understand how to be stewards of other living beings; they learned from their parents, who were likely taught by first generation "off-the-farm" folk. Barn cats and farm dogs were not companion animals, just as the farm horse was not a pleasure horse. Farm dogs got onto the back porch long before barn cats got into the kitchen, but in many rural communities, the barriers to companion animals still exist. If veterinarians do not accept the role of community educator, the animals will suffer.

How does a veterinary healthcare delivery team approach a client who has been neglecting his/her dog, cat, or horse? It should start with a simple, nonthreatening question, followed by sincere listening. A sample question could be, "Do you know there are vaccinations to prevent the barn cat die offs?" It could be, "Do you know we can level that horse's teeth and make winter grazing on feed much more effective?" Or it could even be, "Do you know that the current heartworm medications will also prevent many internal parasites that can be transmitted to kids and cause abdominal flu-like syndrome?" If the veterinarian is assisting local law enforcement officials evaluating a complaint, these questions are not indicated; legal procedures take precedence during the enforcement process.

I have seen animals chained with logging chains, unable to reach water. I have seen animals with hoofs in a full ram's horn curl. I have seen animals with choke chains imbedded in their necks. In each of these cases, the animal owner was basically unaware of the inhumane situation: since their folks had done it, they assumed it was just the way it was. Questions I like to ask take it one step farther: "Would you like to learn about a pet food that would make the litter box smell less?" "Do you know we can restore these hoofs so it does not hurt to walk?" "Would you like to help your pet live a longer life?" Or even, "If we can give your pet good breath, would you like puppy kisses back?" Animal owners who care will ask for more information if the accusations are not personal, if the evaluation comments are based on the environment rather than the personalities, and if the neglect is handled as a lack of education rather than a personal shortcoming.

The Most Difficult of Situations

In the worst case scenario, the animal owner does not care. This is the person who should not have animals, and if the veterinary professional supports the local law enforcement agency, the problem can be addressed. In most every case, a law enforcement official will ask for veterinary assistance when assessing abuse or neglect complaints, and the professional steps should then include:

- Step one. Identify animal neglect in a fair and consistent manner (use Title 9, CFR, and your professional training).
- Step two. Be available for education of law enforcement officials, schools, new pet owners, and people involved in the neglect cases.
- Step three. In the worst case scenario, "neglect" can be elevated to "abuse" when poor treatment through ignorance is replaced by willful harm to an animal. In this case, the veterinary healthcare provider must become an advocate for the animal and accept no compromise in the health, well-being, or quality of life of another living entity.

Our education and experience makes us the experts in evaluating animal welfare; if a veterinarian abdicates this community responsibility, animals suffer, the community suffers, and more importantly, the profession suffers. In life, there are only two basic roles, leader and follower. Leaders develop other people in their daily actions, and animal welfare is one area that makes us feel good when we can make a difference.

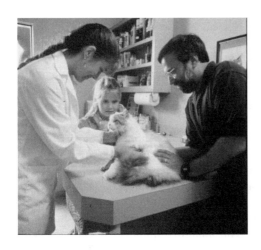

Appendix Z

The "Bond-centered" Practice

SINCE I am a Charter Member of the Delta Society, I was strongly influenced by Dr. Leo Bustad (the true founder of the American human-animal bond movement) from the very beginning of my quest to embrace the bond (over two decades ago). I still remember many of the words he shared, sometimes over a quiet dinner, and more often, when he was promoting the bond in the "early days," when most people did not understand. His passion is what we all need to find, so here are some thoughts Leo wrote in 1988:

For as long as I can remember, I've been thankful I had extensive exposure to a variety of animals and that my parents impressed on me the importance of treating animals gently. During my professional career, I've observed the many benefits that contact with animals has on people of all ages and conditions. As dean of the College of Veterinary Medicine at Washington State University, I studied the significance of animals throughout our society, and I am deeply distressed by the casual disregard for animals' well-being manifested by many people. Irresponsible pet ownership is widespread. I am also disturbed by the lack of behavior training: such training benefits both animals and people in numerous ways.

I realized something had to be done. The relationships between people and animals are important and beautiful. We link ourselves with the world of nature through the animals that share our lives. We marvel at the sheer physical appearance of animals—their eyes, coats, fins, feathers, and their movement. We feel enriched by the obvious pleasure our pets take in our companionship, and we are touched by their sensitivity to our moods. We also derive many practical benefits from our animal companions. In caring for our fellow creatures, we express some of our finest qualities, and it is normal to develop bonds of love with animals that are as powerful as those we experience with people.

In regard to our place on planet Earth, my views, like other authors in the human-animal bond literature, are consistent with those of many Native Americans. I live in the Palouse of eastern Washington and western Idaho—the land of Chief Joseph and the Nez Perce. These ancient Native Americans, who refer to themselves as "The Real People," have a profound comprehension of reality and truth. The word "religion" is not in their vocabulary, for everything has sacred significance. Nature is Mother Earth, and the minerals within her, the vegetation that springs from her, and the animals that roam over her, are sacred. They, along with other groups of enlightened inhabitants of our planet, believe that animals, plants, and the earth are like vital parts of our body—if these parts are compromised, we seriously harm ourselves. To remain healthy, we must maintain a respectful relationship with all the elements of our environment. A strong people-animal-environment bond is crucial to a healthy worldwide community.

The new millennium will see many veterinary practices that claim to be "bond centered." Some will implement the programs listed herein that make them money, but will not change their approach to staff nurturing or veterinary healthcare delivery; these are not "bond-centered" veterinary practices. Some will endorse the Delta Society, join the American Association of Human Animal Bond Veterinarians, and attend all the Vet One meetings, but will not become patient advocates willing to take a stand and tell clients what is needed; these are not "bond-centered" veterinary practices. So where do you start?

The human-animal bond is impacted by the environment, sometimes even with feral and wild animals; we usually cannot control the environment, but we can appreciate the relationship. The human-animal bond is impacted by the community, and there are various areas where a veterinary practice or its professional team can exert its influence [pet population control activities, leash laws and other regulatory interaction, pets by prescription in the school system, humane society support, animal impoundment activities, abuse/neglect expertise (Title 9, CFR), assistance animal support, etc.]. But the major impact of bond-centered practices is as patient advocates delivering client-centered healthcare.

The combination of quality veterinary healthcare delivery programs and a caring heart begins the process, and there is a mixture of steps and elements that must come together to form the bond-centered practice. There are less than a dozen elements in the basic "bond-centered" formula, and they are not listed below in any specific order or priority. The offered list is not all inclusive; it only provides a set of common elements. The expansion beyond these elements is what makes the healthcare delivery of client-centered patient advocacy in any veterinary practice an art and science.

• Understand the quality required in veterinary healthcare delivery, including the *Standards for Veterinary Hospitals* as offered by the American Veterinary Medical Association (this is not the certification, this is the utilization of the *Standards* in daily operations whether you are a member or not). Understand that the leadership, programs, and innovations discussed in *Building the Successful Veterinary Practice* (Catanzaro 1997, 1998) are minimal expectations for practice excellence. Ensure every member of the practice embraces the concepts of patient advocacy, clinical competence, and the celebration of the human-animal-veterinary bond.

• When dealing with others, respect life and respect opinions of others. Do not accept "euthanasia" as an initial treatment in cancer, kidney dysfunction, or chronic care. Understand respite care, hospice, and senior friend screening programs for wellness and support in medically stressful times. To augment your knowledge of thanatology, review chapter 4 of *Healthcare of the Well Pet* (Jevring and Catanzaro, 1998).

• Never allow pain or puking in any patient. We have too many medications available today to allow any patient to "endure pain" or any client to experience recurrent vomiting in their companion animal. Respect the hospital staff, their feelings, and their opinions; monitor their pride as an aspect of the quality of the practice.

• Ensure staff members are assigned responsibilities for outcomes rather than just process. Accept the responsibility for ensuring clients feel good about the treatment modalities, including ensuring they know how and what to feed their companion animals. Don't tell people what *not to do,* tell them what they *can do;* help them learn to help people be winners on their own terms.

• Cease making healthcare "recommendations" to clients. Start clearly stating what is "needed" and learn to then be quiet and listen. When you state what is "needed," write the need with a box, e.g., "X ray ❑" (instead of "recommend X ray"). Then, after listening, enter the client's response in the box: W = waiver, D = defer, A = appointment, and X = do it! After and "D" or "A," enter the time until the recheck, e.g. X ray ☒ 72h (as in, ". . . if the limp has not resolved in three days, I need you to bring Spike back in for the X rays!").

• Become an advocate of quality preventive healthcare, including "over 40" physicals (anthropomorphic comparisons are permitted and encouraged). The "over 40" physical is a well-known healthcare standard in human healthcare in the United States and should become equally well accepted in companion animal care (Canada does not publicize it as well due to the access limitation encountered with socialized healthcare programs). For veterinary practices, this "over 40" physical includes thoracic X rays, abdominal X rays, CBC, blood chemistry profile, ECG, and breed-specific needs (e.g., thyroid and blood pressure in cats, gout in Dalmatians, ocular pressure in "bug eyed" dogs, etc.). Also, the bond-centered practice will stand for standards of excellence, such as pain scoring, body scoring, dental scoring, nutritional scoring, preanesthetic blood screens, preanesthetic risk assessments, vaccine protection, flea and tick protection, zoonotic disease screens (e.g., fecals and blood tests), and annual life-cycle consultations, which include traveling with your pet and assessment of nutritional needs.

- Never quit learning, personally or as a practice. Never defer educating clients in becoming better stewards of living entities; clients need professional assistance in learning these new skills. Embrace and support continuing education for the practice staff. This includes distance learning for staff members who want to become "certified" in their disciplines (e.g., CVT/RVT/LVT for technicians, CVPM for managers, etc.) . Strive to find new ways to extend the quality of life of all living things, including Subchapter A, Chapter 1, Title 9, Code of Federal Regulations (implementation of the Animal Welfare Act). Never quit striving for the next level of excellence.
- Manage the veterinary practice from the heart (Bracey et al. 1990):

    H = Hear and understand the team members.
    E = Even if you disagree, don't make them wrong.
    A = Acknowledge the greatness within each person.
    R = Remember to look for their caring intentions.
    T = Tell them the truth with compassion.

- Give recognition, specifically and regularly, so appropriate behavior will be repeated (behavior rewarded is behavior repeated). Appreciate the quest for a balanced life by healthcare providers, and recognize individual contributions for performance during realistic shifts, not excessive duty hours.
- Last, but not the least important, is the tone and feel of the practice. When we celebrate the bond, we are celebrating the ability to enhance the quality of life of a family member within a stewardship. Every staff member is empowered to embrace opportunities to enhance the quality of life; every patient has the right to access the best veterinary care; and every provider speaks for the needs of the animal at every opportunity. Clients are treated as stewards of living entities who want the best for their family member; healthcare and wellness decisions are not made unilaterally by the practice team.

As the human-animal bond increases the value of the pet in the family, there are inherent and concurrent impacts. Courts may start to award "pain and suffering" findings against veterinary practices who do not fully inform clients of the consequence of the healthcare delivery decisions. In human healthcare, informed consent seldom includes protection for the provider who allows clients to defer or refuse care; courts have found that clients do not have adequate knowledge to be allowed to put themselves into that position of jeopardy. Healthcare standards at veterinary facilities will rise as a systemic expectation, including more aggressive pain management, fluid therapy during most all surgeries (e.g., IV TKO—To Keep Open), and preanesthetic blood screening; the lack of these programs in a practice's standard delivery will become a liability. The trend will increase the cost of veterinary healthcare, so pet health insurance use probably will increase (some European communities are already seeing in excess of 50 percent pet population insurance coverage). Practices will no longer be able to offer coupons and cut corners (or do "bait and switch" sales), nor will they just absorb the cost of higher quality healthcare; veterinary practices will need to share the value of services with the stewards of pets and charge accordingly.

The bond-centered practice may not be well defined in the veterinary profession or the family household, but when clients experience it, they know they have discovered something special. The bond-centered practice can be the differentiation in the community that builds the word-of-mouth reputation, but that is not its primary goal; it is just an additional outcome. The bond-centered practice does not ask, "What's in it for me" as an initial assessment, but concurrently, it charges appropriate fees for the exemplary services it provides; we see a referral by word-of-mouth in excess of the magic 60 percent of all new client transactions.

The bond-centered practice is not for everyone; some staff and some clients will not "get it." Many people were raised with "barn cats" and "farm dogs," and their basic values do not include patient advocacy for all animals; accept this diversity in the population and be happy when they seek another practice to visit. The bond-centered practice embraces the opportunity to offer a special environment for staff and clients who want to experience patient-advocate healthcare delivery. The client-centered services of a bond-centered practice listen to the client and allow for joint, rather than unilateral, healthcare decisions; the practice does not mandate or abdicate in the joint decision process.

The bond-centered practice is a wonder to behold; it provides a very special feeling to all who enter. Interaction between clients, veterinarians, and staff in such a practice creates an appreciation of the family-pet-veterinary bond; the bond-centered practice also fosters an increased awareness of people-animals-environment relationships. This reference text is the beginning, not the end, of discussions about "how to get there" in a practice team that cares enough to become a bond-centered leader in the veterinary profession, community, and greater healthcare delivery system.

References

Bracey, H., J. Rosenblum, A. Sanford, and R. Trueblood (Contributor). 1990. *Managing from the Heart.* New York: Delacorte Press.

Catanzaro, T.E. 1997. *Building the Successful Veterinary Practice: Leadership Tools.* Ames: Iowa State University Press.

Catanzaro, T.E. 1998. *Building the Successful Veterinary Practice: Programs and Procedures.* Ames: Iowa State University Press.

Catanzaro, T.E. 1998. *Building the Successful Veterinary Practice: Innovation and Creativity.* Ames: Iowa State University Press.

Jevring, C., and T.E. Catanzaro. 1998. *Healthcare of the Well Pet.* Bailliere-Tindale.

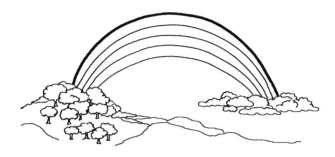

The Rainbow Bridge

There is a bridge connecting Heaven and Earth. It is called the Rainbow Bridge because of its many colors. Just this side of the Rainbow Bridge there is a land of meadows, hills and valleys with lush green grass.

When a beloved pet dies, the pet goes to this place. There is always food and water and warm spring weather. The old and frail animals are young again. Those who are maimed are made whole again. They play all day with each other.

There is only one thing missing. They are not with the special person who loved them on Earth. So, each day they run and play until the day comes when one suddenly stops playing and looks up! The nose twitches! The ears up! The eyes are staring! And this one suddenly runs from the group!

You have been seen, and when you and your special friend meet, you take him or her in you arms and embrace. Your face is kissed again and again, and you look once more into the eyes of your trusting pet.

Then you cross the Rainbow Bridge together, never again to be separated.

—Author Unknown